Contents

Contents

About the author

Dr John Mansfield has been working in the field of food sensitivity since 1976, when he became one of three original British pioneers. In 1978 he was a founder member of the British Society for Allergy and Environmental Medicine and became its President from 1992 to 1995. He gained his medical degree at Guy's Hospital, London, and has worked in both the UK and the USA. He has written a number of best-selling health books, including *The Migraine Revolution, Arthritis – the allergy connection,* and *The Asthma Epidemic.*

Acknowledgements

First of all, I shall always be grateful to the physicians who guided and influenced me in the early days of my career in this subject. They include Dr Richard Mackarness, who introduced me to this fascinating area of medicine. From England there were also Professor Ronald Finn, Dr Stephen Davies and Professor Jonathan Brostoff, and many others too numerous to mention. From the USA there were Dr Theron Randolph, Professor William Rea and Professor Joseph Miller.

In preparing this book I would particularly like to thank Dr Shideh Pouria for her help with some areas and for many general interesting discussions. Mrs Eve Forbes kindly proof read the manuscript for me before it was delivered to the publisher, for which I would like to thank her.

Finally, and most of all, I would like to thank my wife Diane for constantly pointing out whenever I strayed into unnecessary detail as she constantly typed and retyped each chapter. She also pointed out (by yawning!) whenever I lapsed into overly scientific (boring?) terminology.

Foreword

More and more people are struggling with achieving their ideal weight today. Obesity and weight problems have reached epidemic proportions in the western world in the last decade. The repetitive mantra of the doctors, dieticians and governments is to reduce caloric intake and increase exercise. Yet this approach has not produced the desired results. The experts are stuck in the narrow one-track conceptual groove of calorie control despite this strategy consistently failing millions of people, and despite much evidence against it.

Why did obesity rates double in one decade (the 1980s) in countries such as the US and the UK where people systematically cut out fats from their diets, and increased their levels of exercise? Why are the French still the slimmest people in Europe despite their very high dietary fat intake?

This book offers a different perspective and radical alternatives to the inertia that has beset the 'diet industry' and the medical and dietetic professions in dealing with weight problems. It answers the questions above and many more with the kind of lateral thinking that we have come to expect from Dr John Mansfield. At a time when the medical profession can only come up with more of the same, he has provided real, practical and working solutions based on years of experience as one of the pioneers of ecological medicine in this country.

Dr Mansfield and other doctors working in the fields of allergy, environmental and nutritional medicine have been successfully treating patients using approaches that are personalised to the patient rather than the ineffective one-size-fits-all. The observation that many other processes may affect the control of weight has paved the way for a more comprehensive approach. This includes investigation of the role of food intolerances, imbalances in the bacteria residing in the mucus membranes of the gastrointestinal tract, hormonal imbalance, and others. Many patients treated in this way have avoided the lifetime of misery and poor health ensuing from the low-calorie, low-fat diets that don't work.

I had the good fortune of coming across Dr Mansfield and his colleagues while working as a consultant at Guy's Hospital, as a result of trying to help a colleague with similar intractable problems and no hope of regaining her health. What he did in that case, and in many subsequent cases with which I became involved after I left Guy's, was often described by his patients as being nothing short of miraculous.

These extraordinary stories stem from the fact that he was, and remains, one of the leading medical thinkers who have dared to think outside the box in the interest of healing and alleviating suffering in his patients. I cannot recommend this book highly enough for those seeking intelligent and more effective solutions to their weight problems.

Dr Shideh Pouria
MB BS BSc MRCP(UK) PhD CMT

Chapter 1

What is this book all about?

This book is dedicated to the millions of people who are over-weight, to a lesser or greater extent, because they are being given the wrong medical advice and so eating the wrong foods. Poor advice is not the only reason for not achieving your ideal weight. There are very genuine reasons why people put on weight, and they are not about eating too much.

Dear Reader, you may be one of the many well-motivated, but nevertheless overweight people who have diligently followed various diets for years. You may have seen initial weight reduction, but in general your weight has steadily increased year after year despite your best efforts. You are not alone. People who struggle with their weight are often perceived as weak willed. A few may be; many are anything but and have achieved much in their lives. You may be surprised to learn that both low-calorie and low-fat diets can actually promote an increase in weight in the long term. This is why the inhabitants of the countries that follow them most closely have become the fattest on the planet.

Many people still think the cause of weight gain is simply eating too many calories, and so the solution is therefore merely to eat fewer calories and burn more through exercise. How nice it would be if it were that simple. If it was, the USA, UK and Mexico would probably be the three slimmest nations in the world, as nowhere else has had more advice on how to reduce calories and fat. Instead, these are the three fattest nations, with Americans eating the lowest-fat diet in the western world, while being by far the fattest nation.

The first secret

Avoiding low-calorie diets is the first secret of successful weight loss. Low-calorie diets are a particularly unsuccessful way of treating weight problems as they are not addressing any specific cause of weight gain. They are really treating a symptom and not a fundamental cause, like treating back pain with painkillers. The back pain may be caused by a disc problem, misaligned intervertebral joints or many other conditions. Dealing with the cause usually eradicates the problem, while taking painkillers could be an unsatisfactory lifetime sentence.

Furthermore, low-calorie diets activate certain basic survival mechanisms that protected our Stone Age ancestors from the frequent threat of starvation when food supplies were scarce. These mechanisms include increasing our insulation and decreasing our metabolic rate. They click into action on low-calorie diets and explain why reduced calorie intake can initially be successful, but weight loss grinds to a halt in a few weeks. The details of these mechanisms and the sequence of events they lead to are described in the next chapter. Countless people have been driven to distraction on these diets. They are, in fact, a form of semi-starvation and consequently one of the most elegant forms of mental and physical torture ever devised.

The second secret

The second secret of successful weight loss then is to avoid low-fat diets. You may have been following one in the belief that it will protect you from developing heart disease in the future. This is far from the truth. The theory about the adverse effects of cholesterol is totally flawed, and has not led to any reduction in deaths from coronary artery disease. The reduction that has been seen correlates with the massive reduction in cigarette smoking.

Chapter 9 is called 'The cholesterol myth and why low-fat diets are a major cause of weight gain'. For over 40 years, I have followed the amazing twists and turns of the theory that eating cholesterol is harmful. Much of this theory is reminiscent of the fable of the *Emperor's New Clothes*. The science supporting it has been completely invalidated (see pages 146-9), yet 'low fat' labelling continues and the health of hundreds of millions of people worldwide is directly affected. The theory has now been disowned even by its originator, Professor Ancel Keys. As long ago as 1997 he stated: 'There is no connection between cholesterol in food and cholesterol in the blood, and we have known this all along. Cholesterol in the diet does not matter at all unless you happen to be a chicken or rabbit.'

The real causes of coronary artery disease have become increasingly more obvious in the past decade or so and are discussed in chapters 10 to 12. All that low-fat diets have achieved is to treble the incidence of clinical obesity.

The year 1980 played a very significant role in the history of the USA and UK. The year marked the start of a dramatic increase in clinical obesity on both sides of the Atlantic. A year or so earlier the American people had been told that they should severely reduce saturated fat (or cholesterol) in their diet. Britain quickly followed suit. By 1980, the majority of American and British people had reduced the amount of fat they ate. The next 11 years from 1980 to 1991 saw the incidence of clinical obesity double in both nations, and this trend continued so that by 2005 the incidence had trebled.* By contrast the two decades preceding1980 had seen no appreciable rise at all.

Now I have told you what not to do I will reveal the secrets of what you *should* do. **This book's unique approach is that it**

*There is a vast quantity of medical literature describing the consequences of the change to low-fat diets. The UK statistics quoted here were published in the *British Medical Journal* in 1995.

looks at your weight gain as a condition that has causes specific to you that can be discovered. They can then be successfully dealt with, leading to a return to your ideal weight.

The third secret

The third secret of successful weight loss is to find out if you are sensitive to any ordinary, everyday foods. Food sensitivities, which vary considerably from one person to another, are by far the commonest single cause of weight gain. They were the prime cause in more than 70% of the patients I treated over a period of 31 years in clinical practice, specialising in Allergy and Nutritional Medicine. In 1976, I started to investigate food sensitivity as a cause of various illnesses. My first few patients were also decidedly overweight. I put them all on my elimination diet. This diet (described in chapter 5) is a collection of around 40 foods that are highly unlikely to cause any problems. These can be eaten while avoiding all foods that commonly are a problem for seven days. My first patient lost 11 lb (5 kg) and all of her symptoms in those first seven days. She then reintroduced single foods, one at each meal, and was able to identify just three foods that were the root of all her problems. In three months her weight dropped from 13 stone 2 lb (184 lb or 83.5 kg) to her original weight of 8 stone 12 lb (124 lb or 56 kg). When I last saw her seven years later she still weighed the same and had had no recurrence of her medical condition. I realised I had stumbled across an actual cause of weight gain, as there had been absolutely no calorie restriction whatsoever. I was actually blown away by this turn of events. Was she just a one in a million fluke? The next eight patients all responded in the same way, so it was obviously a common factor which I now know solves weight and other medical problems in nearly three quarters of people.

Chapter 3 describes in detail what happened when five patients went on my elimination diet. Case histories are a very good way of explaining what food sensitivity is all about. Chapter 4 explains all you need to know about what food sensitivity is, so you can understand what is happening as you go through each stage of the elimination diet.

As I've said, the diet itself is described in detail in chapter 5. This chapter, for most people, will be the most important one in the book, and contains a step-by-step account of how to follow this diet. I know of no single strategy in medicine that has changed more people's lives than this simple diet. Please do not be tempted to do blood tests which are usually inaccurate and very expensive.

If you are interested in using the technique of desensitisation to your food sensitivities, I have described it in detail in chapter 6. This technique enables you to eat foods already identified as causing problems on the elimination diet, without weight gain or symptoms. This method is vital to the unlucky few who have multiple food sensitivities or sensitivities to foods that are very difficult to avoid.

We should now consider the three remaining secrets of successful weight loss by looking at other causes of weight gain. These are the 'yeast syndrome', persistently high blood levels of insulin (hyperinsulinaemia), and low output of thyroid hormone (hypothyroidism). If you feel you have achieved your ideal weight by sorting out any food sensitivities then there is obviously no need to bother with looking at these. If, however, you feel you have more weight you would like to lose, or food sensitivity does not appear to be the cause for you, it is then worthwhile looking at these other areas.

The fourth secret

So chapter 7 covers the fourth secret of successful weight loss: treating, if necessary, the yeast syndrome (also known as the '*Candida* problem'). In this condition there is an overgrowth of naturally occurring yeasts in the gut which can produce toxins. These toxins can interfere with your weight regulating mechanisms in a similar way to food sensitivity. It is probably the third most common cause of weight gain after food sensitivity and low-fat diets. It can be diagnosed by the presence of certain symptoms and a useful, but optional, blood test. The treatment consists of an appropriate diet and anti-yeast preparations. There is a questionnaire in chapter 14 to help you determine if you have this problem.

The fifth secret

The fifth secret to successful weight loss is correcting hyperinsulinaemia. Hyperinsulinaemia is the medical term for persistently high levels of insulin in the blood. In chapter 10 I explain how, in fact, it is insulin that is largely responsible for laying down fat. It does this by converting refined carbohydrates directly to fat. Eating fat does not lead to excess fat, but eating refined carbohydrates does. This condition is especially common in people who are very overweight. Chapter 10 is entitled, 'How refined carbohydrates cause weight gain and health problems'. These carbohydrates were not available in any great quantity until after the 1850s. Over the past 160 years the consumption of these foods has risen, gradually at first, but dramatically later. The incidence of weight gain, diabetes and coronary artery disease matches this rise. I explain in chapter 10 the precise reasons why this has happened.

Chapter 12 ties together a lot of the themes from the preceding three chapters. It relates how some weight problems, and all cases of diabetes and coronary heart disease, are fundamentally a man-made disaster. This originates from thoughtless decisions, made around 160 years ago, to modify extensively staple foods that form a major part of our diet.

The sixth secret

The final, sixth, secret of successful weight loss is to investigate the possibility of hypothyroidism. This refers to the low production of thyroid hormones from the thyroid gland, and is covered in chapter 8. This is a well-recognised cause of weight gain and has been known as such for many decades. The management of this condition is not dietary and involves the use of thyroid hormones. Consequently, it needs to be managed by a doctor.

The subject of exercise is covered in chapter 13. I think exercise is vital for good health, but exercise alone is not enough to make you lose weight, unless you are young and only mildly overweight. A lack of exercise is not a major cause of weight problems. In a nutshell, it is difficult for exercise to counteract a fundamental cause of weight gain, such as food sensitivity. Chapter 13 includes some interesting studies on the long-term effect of heavy exercise on weight management.

Chapter 14 provides a step-by-step guide to how you can identify the cause/s of your own weight gain, including two useful questionnaires. This will help you to put into practice what you have learned throughout the book.

I sincerely hope that this book changes your life for the better and that you no longer have to endure the utter frustration of low-calorie diets with their attendant problems of persistent hunger and fatigue. I promise there is no place in this book where you are advised to limit the quantity of food that you eat. You just need to eat the foods that are right for *you*.

This book is about empowerment. If you discover the root cause of your weight problems you will, at last, have control of your weight and be enabled to remain fit and healthy for the rest of your life.

Chapter 2

Why low-calorie diets do NOT work in the long term

It has been reported that, at any one time, 50% of the adult population of the UK are 'on a diet'. These diets are usually low- calorie or low-fat diets in different guises. People very frequently emerge from the experience frustrated, bewildered, angry and very disappointed.

On 27 September 2007 the *Daily Mail* in its *Femail Magazine* section made the following statement:

> '*As we become the world's 3rd fattest nation one diet coach asks "Why do slimmers always get fat?"*'

In this article, Sally Ann Voak, one of Britain's most prolific slimming writers, whose 28 books have sold over a million copies, acknowledged: 'I have failed in my almost evangelical mission to slim the nation'. Like most diet books, Sally Ann's advocate reducing calories and fat while increasing exercise, yet as she says: 'I know now that over 60 per cent of the many people I have slimmed have put back some (in some cases all) of the weight they once carried.'

In my view, she and many millions of low calorie-dieters have been badly misled and 'sold a pup' by a medical profession slavishly following a dangerously simplistic view of what causes people to become overweight.

If the low-calorie diet approach was successful, the USA and Great Britain would be the slimmest nations on Earth! In these countries all the media portray slimness in both females and males as the ideal form. Sally Ann Voak says she has yet to meet a really happy fat person. Nobody likes looking in the mirror and seeing a fat body. It is impossible to carry a large amount of weight with all the limitations it entails and be truly happy with yourself.

The truth is that in the short term, low calorie diets can be quite successful, but in the long run they make the problem much worse than not dieting at all; I will describe the reasons for this in just a moment.

The calorific principle of dieting was originally described in 1930 by two doctors, Dr Newburgh and Dr Johnson.[2] Working at the University of Michigan in the USA, they thought that if we consume fewer calories than our bodies burn, we are bound to lose weight. They said that if our bodies burn 2000 calories a day, but we consume 1500 calories a day, we will have a deficit of 500 calories. To compensate for this our bodies will burn stored fuel and we will lose weight. However, in reality, the calorie control principle is dangerously simplistic.

Human beings, like animals, have very sophisticated biological systems to protect them from periods of starvation, which were very common when our hunter gatherer ancestors were unable to find enough food, especially during winter months in Northern Europe. These weight conservation mechanisms consist of two different complementary strategies:

- increasing the insulation of the body;
- lowering the basal metabolic rate – the speed at which the body keeps working.

Increasing insulation

We have two types of fat cells:

- white fat cells;
- brown fat cells.

White fat cells are present in the layer immediately under the skin known as the subcutaneous space, and in situations of semi-starvation, such as occur in low calorie diets, increased white fat cells form to conserve energy. Thus a mechanism which saved our ancestors from dying of starvation can thwart periods of controlled semi-starvation now - that is, low-calorie diets.

Brown fat cells, in contrast, are located mostly in the thoracic cavity (chest) attached to long blood vessels along the back and shoulder bones. They are also present in the armpits and the nape of the neck.

About 10–15% of total fat is composed of brown fat cells while 85–90% is composed of white fat cells. The presence of brown fat cells was discovered by scientists investigating the ability of hibernating bears to maintain a persistently high body temperature throughout the winter. Apparently the large store of brown fat stimulated by the cold temperature enables the bears to keep their heat production high. Thus brown fat cells burn excess calories to produce body heat whereas white fat cells mostly store it. Overweight people seem to have less activated brown fat than thin people and as a consequence lower overall metabolism.

A thin person with a good supply of efficiently functioning brown fat can thus convert extra calories into body heat and not gain weight when overeating. The fat person, on the same calorie diet, eventually gains weight by storing the extra calories as white fat. One way to help weight problems to some extent is to stimulate brown fat metabolism with the help of essential fatty acids such as evening primrose oil in particular and fish oils to a lesser extent.

Another issue to contend with is that when you starve yourself on a low-calorie diet your supply of an important enzyme – cell membrane lipoprotein lipase (LPL) – increases by something like seven to 40 times. An enzyme is a substance produced by the body that enables chemical reactions to take place. This enzyme draws blood fats (triglycerides) from the blood into the white fat cells for storage. The more those calories are restricted, the more efficient this mechanism becomes. What this means is the more you restrict your calorie intake, the easier it is for you subsequently to gain weight. In fact, it can be up to 40 times easier.

The classic stages of low-calorie dieting

Lipoprotein lipase activity is mostly controlled by the hormone insulin.[3] Sex hormones such as testosterone, oestrogen and progesterone also play some part in the process. Insulin has also been described as the 'gatekeeper' hormone for fat accumulation. In fatty tissues, insulin increases LPL activity but in the muscles it decreases it. Thus when insulin levels rise, more fat is deposited in fatty tissues and less is available for the muscles to burn to produce energy. When insulin levels drop the opposite occurs.

Women have more LPL activity in their adipose (fatty) tissue than men. When one considers the change in the distribution of fat in the body as people age, sex hormones play a part in both sexes. In men there is more LPL activity in the upper abdomen accounting for the classic 'beer belly'. This LPL activity is kept in check by high levels of testosterone when men are young. As testosterone levels gradually fall the rising levels of LPL activity cause the 'beer belly' to become worse. Women have more LPL activity in their hips and buttocks regulated by progesterone. However, similar to men, high levels of oestrogen check the LPL activity in the abdomen. Oestrogen levels decrease during and after the menopause and this reduction increases LPL activity in the abdomen. Hence women accumulate more fat in that area post menopause.

Very importantly, research has shown that LPL activity in fatty tissues increases when weight loss occurs as a result of calorie restriction. Conversely, in muscle tissue LPL activity decreases, explaining the muscle wasting seen in severe calorie-restricted diets. These changes do not occur with diets that only restrict carbohydrates.

Reduction in metabolic rate

We now come to the body's reduction in metabolic rate, the body's other response to starvation. Whenever there is a sudden decrease in calorie consumption, our bodies adjust our metabolic rate downwards. You can test this by taking your temperature. Often, mid-morning temperature under the tongue will show a reduction of about 2° Fahrenheit (96.5° F (35.8°C) as opposed to 98.4° F (36.9°C)) when the metabolic 'fire' reduces. This occurs because there is insufficient fuel to feed it and the metabolic rate decreases to save what fuel there is.

When you eventually stop depriving yourself it takes some time for your body to catch on that it has increased its intake by, say, 1000 calories per day. These extra calories have nowhere to go and so are now stored as white fat. Eventually your body's thermostat catches on and burns more calories, but not before a huge weight gain has occurred.

Furthermore, restricted calorie intake leads to other negative consequences. Immune function and adrenal gland activity reduce and the body becomes malnourished. It cannot possibly get adequate nutrients on a daily diet of 600–1200 calories. Essentially, the lack of fibre, vitamins, minerals, amino acids and essential fatty acids will lead to poor health in all its various manifestations.

These responses to calorie restriction are just some of the mechanisms involved in the disastrous long-term effects of low calorie dieting.

There is a standard sequence of events which occurs and affects almost every low-calorie dieter, and answers Sally Ann Voaks' question: 'Why do slimmers always get fat, or should we say, get fatter?'

At first, low-calorie diets seem to be very effective, and lots of weight disappears, depending on how much needs to be lost and how restrictive the diet. At this point one could say that it 'flatters to deceive'. Soon the body realises that it appears to be starving, and the usual mechanisms of increasing insulation and decreasing metabolic rate start to click in. As this happens, the rate of weight loss slows fairly quickly to nothing.

After a week or so of no further weight loss, the dieter understandably becomes frustrated. What usually happens at this point is that the person goes to a social event and because of the frustration, breaks the diet, often quite spectacularly. S/he regains a significant amount of the lost weight in a few days, maybe even reaching a weight level higher than the original starting level. Even with strict adherence to the diet, some people will still gain weight eventually.

The dieter has thus gone through the standard three stages classically seen in low-calorie diets and already listed above: weight loss, stabilisation (when no further weight is lost), and weight gain. After licking his/her wounds, the dieter then decides to try a stricter diet (500 fewer calories) but does not manage to get down to the weight lost on the original diet. The same sequence of weight loss and weight stabilisation followed by weight gain occurs. Again the weight gain often exceeds the weight gain of the first attempt.

This is referred to, in newspapers and magazines, as 'Yo-Yo dieting' and is much frowned upon. However, it is an almost inevitable consequence of the low-calorie dieting.

Thus a person with what may be a minor weight problem can be converted to a person with a major weight problem in as short a time as three or four years. In this way, calorie-controlled diets are not only ineffective, but can become, in some people, an important **cause** of obesity.

Countless people have been through this sequence of events and have emerged battered and bruised and usually fatter. Many of them have said to me: 'I have been on countless diets and each one has eventually made me worse.' These diets are, I hasten to add, calorie-control diets only.

The conventional view is that obese people eat too much and

sometimes this is true, but a recent French study showed that:

- only 15% of obese people eat too much (2800–4000 calories daily)
- 35% of obese people eat normally (2000–2700 calories daily)
- 50% of obese people eat less (800–1500 calories daily).

Think of the miserable lives that 50% of obese people live – despite being on a very restricted diet they remain clinically obese. Such studies confirm that low-calorie diets don't work.

The inevitable consequence of muscle wasting

There is no dispute that all low-calorie diets inevitably lead to some degree of muscle wasting. Apart from the undesirable appearance of this, the main problem is that muscle mass is a major factor in the burning of calories, so by losing muscle mass your ability to burn calories will be further diminished.

Evidence for the failure of low-calorie diets

One of the few physicians who have looked objectively at low-calorie diets was Dr Albert Stunkard at the New York Hospital. He had been struck by the fact that he had had great problems in getting patients to slim with low-calorie diets, when there was a general assumption that it was all relatively straightforward. He scoured the medical literature and managed to find eight studies that led to accurate assessment of whether low-calorie or semi-starvation diets (which is what they used to be called) were effective.

All of these studies used greatly obese patients for assessment. Only 25% of the patients studied lost over 20 lb (9 kg) and only 5% lost 40 lb (18 kg), though these were only relatively small losses for such grossly obese people.

Dr Stunkard then undertook his own study[4] of 100 patients limited to between 800 and 1500 calories a day. Of these people, only 12% were able to lose 20 lb (9 kg) and just one person lost 40 lb (18 kg).

The thing that really matters in all of these studies is how many successes were still present after one or two years. In the Stunkard study, only two patients out of the original 100 had managed to maintain their weight loss after this time. He concluded that the adverse effects caused by low-calorie diets outweighed any minimal benefit. This conclusion has also been reached by numerous other doctors and countless patients that I have met over many years in practice.

In 2002, a large group of eminent scientists gathered to assess all the evidence relating to the success or otherwise of low-calorie and low-fat diets. This procedure of assessing all the published evidence on a medical issue became known as a Cochrane Collaboration. The outcome was that they considered that low-fat diets produced no more weight loss than low-calorie diets, and in both cases the weigh loss achieved was so small as to be clinically insignificant.

Finally, the UK government statistics (see Figure 2.1) have shown, as described in the first chapter, that the number of calories we eat has steadily decreased. Also the percentage of those calories derived from fat has steadily decreased. Yet the percentage of obese people has steadily increased. Despite all this evidence, books on slimming advocating low-fat low-calorie diets continue to sell and similar diets are handed out in hospital outpatient departments. Low-fat diets are perhaps the biggest disaster of all. I have devoted the whole of chapters 9 and 10 to explaining exactly why this is.

My diets do NOT restrict quantities

Later in this book I explain why identifying food sensitivities is fundamental in sorting out the basic causes of weight problems. It should be noted that calories are not mentioned at any time in chapter 5 on elimination diets. Patients even on the most restrictive part of my elimination diet – stage one, which lasts for only seven days – will usually eat somewhere between 2000 and 3000

Figure 2.1: UK government statistics show that although the percentage of obese people is rapidly increasing, at the same time the number of calories eaten has steadily decreased.

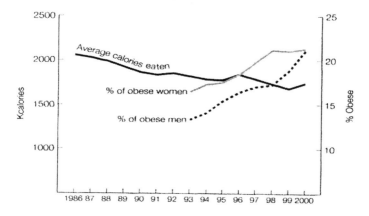

calories a day, depending on their specific choice of which foods to consume. Later on, during stages two and three, when the number of foods allowed increases quickly, the potential calorie content increases further.

Weight loss, often spectacular, in the first seven days (stage one) is due to the elimination of food sensitivities and not to low calorific intake. The same applies in the chapters on the yeast problem.

Reading the current chapter you may recognise your own experience of the effects of low-calorie dieting. You may be curious to know how you can reverse the lowered metabolic rate and increased insulation before you embark on one of the strategies described in this book. I suggest that for three weeks you eat three meals a day of good quality food, as described in chapter 14. This will not have any immediate benefit for your weight, but it will set your metabolism back to normal.

Chapter summary

- Millions of people who have tried countless variations of low-calorie dieting have given up. To back up their personal experience, there is good evidence from clinical trials that low-calorie diets are a disaster in the long term.

- In periods of calorie deprivation, the body concludes that it is being starved and increases its insulation and decreases its metabolic rate to prevent further weight loss.
- **Insulation is increased** as a result of the white fat cells just under the skin increasing in number and the enzyme cell membrane lipoprotein lipase (LPL) being produced in much larger quantities, drawing blood fats (triglycerides) from the blood into the white fat cells for storage.
- **Body metabolism is reduced** by the body slowing down to conserve energy, which can be witnessed by a reduced body temperature of as much as $2°$ F ($1.1°$ C) mid-morning.
- Thus the more you restrict calories, the easier it is for you to gain weight when you start to eat normally again.
- The stages that follow the start of a low-calorie diet are:
  o weight loss
  o weight stabilisation (when no further weight is lost)
  o weight gain (when weight gain often exceeds the person's weight before the diet was started).
- As a result, repeated attempts at low-calorie dieting can lead to increased periods of weight gain, ending up as an important *cause* of obesity.
- Chapter 14 describes the best way to correct the adverse effects of low-calorie and low-fat dieting before you embark on the elimination diet (chapter 5).

Chapter 3

People with food sensitivities causing weight problems: five case histories

In April 1976 I met a British doctor called Dr Richard Mackarness and it changed my whole approach to medicine. I had heard him talk on the radio about his book called *Not All in the Mind* which had been published that day. The theme of the book was that sensitivity, intolerance or allergy to individual foods was the fundamental cause of a lot of ill health. The foods involved were usually commonly consumed ones like the various cereal grains, yeast, eggs, soy, coffee, tea, cane sugar, beet sugar and potatoes. As these foods were consumed daily the patients rarely, if ever, noticed a link between eating them and their symptoms. Dr Mackarness was a consultant psychiatrist so a number of the case histories in his book were of people suffering from depression, although other conditions were also included.

I was fascinated by what he said and rang him to discuss the subject. He invited me to his clinic at Basingstoke General Hospital. A few days later I attended this clinic, accompanied by my trainee, to observe him treating his patients (both in-patients and outpatients) with eliminations diets – very restricted short-term diets after which foods are individually re-introduced to see which are causing problems. The results were spectacular in many patients suffering from fairly wide ranges of symptoms. One of these symptoms was being overweight.

I have detailed below five representative examples of patients I have seen over the last 32 years at my clinic. Over those years I have developed and refined my elimination diet to help people successfully identify foods to which they have been reacting adversely, with minimal inconvenience and cost. It must be emphasised that this is a diet about WHAT you eat, NOT about how much you eat. You can eat as much as you like of the permitted foods at each stage, as described in chapter 5.

Case history 1: Jennifer C

The first patient I ever put on an elimination diet myself was Jennifer C. I had treated Jennifer for over six years in my NHS/private practice. When I saw her in late April 1976 I was very concerned about how she was progressing. The reason for this was that despite six years of antidepressant therapy and visits to various psychiatrists, her depression was worse than ever. Furthermore, she was gaining weight at an alarming rate. When she had got married 15 years before, at the age of 23, her weight had been 8 stone 12 lb (124 lb or 56 kg), her height meanwhile being 5 feet 6 inches (1.68 metres). The combination of rapid weight gain and depression was similar to several patients I had seen at Dr Mackarness's clinic so I elected to take her off her antidepressants and put her on an elimination diet.

She was asked to restrict her diet considerably. With experience I have been able to expand the number of foods allowed on the first stage of the diet to 40, making it far nicer to follow, but without losing any of its effectiveness. Jennifer had a much more limited range available at this early stage. I confirmed that her weight was 13 stone 2 lb (184 lb or 83.5 kg), and explained that it was predicted that the first few days on the diet might make her feel considerably worse. The reasons for this I will explain in the next chapter, but to put it simply, a withdrawal reaction is to be expected when food sensitivity is present.

On the first few days of the diet, particularly the second and third, Jennifer felt very depressed and I called her each day to check on how she was, and to encourage her to continue. However, by day five she was definitely feeling much improved so I waited till day seven before I saw her. On day seven, she was laughing and giggling and her eyes were shining. I had never seen her so well or happy; furthermore, she had lost 11 lb (5 kg) in the seven days, which pleased her even more. In my 12 years of experience in general practice I had never seen such a trans-formation in a patient within a period as short as seven days. Her weight had reduced from the original 13 stone 2 lb (184 lb or 83.5 kg) to 12 stone 5 lb (173 lb or 78.5 kg). Subsequent experience in this area told me that the loss of 11 lb (5 kg) weight on a 'safe' diet could only mean that her weight problem was caused by food sensitivity.

I then suggested various foods that she should introduce one at each meal, with at least five hours between meals. In other words she could test three new foods each day – that is, one at breakfast, one at lunch and one at dinner. At first I suggested she tried foods that I thought there was a good chance she would be perfectly fine with, like green beans, chicken, broccoli, melon and rice. On these foods Jennifer continued to feel really well and continued to lose weight at a rate of approximately 3–4 lb (1.5–2 kg) per week

When she added tomatoes to her list of safe foods, within 2-3 hours she started to feel very depressed again and to her horror she gained 2.5 lb (1 kg) in weight, also within a few hours. She obviously discontinued the tomatoes and carried on eating the safe foods for the next 36 hours, during which time she lost the depression and the weight gain that had occurred as a result of eating the tomatoes. She then continued to lose weight and feel well as other new foods were added.

About five days later she added potatoes to her diet and experienced the same reaction as she had done with tomatoes. I explained to her that potatoes and tomatoes are both in the same food group, known as the solenacia or deadly nightshade family. A few days later she started to introduce the various cereal grains, sugars and such like. They react more slowly than other foods, particularly the cereal grains, so I asked Jennifer to try just one grain for three meals a day for two days. Wheat, oats and rye produced no reaction at all for Jennifer, but corn did. Again the reaction was depression and weight gain. Corn is found, of course, in corn-on-the-cob, but corn flour, corn oil and glucose are all derived from corn and have the same sensitivity type response. These are present in a wide range of foods like cakes, biscuits and gravy and are used as a thickener in an extensive range of processed foods. Corn, often being 'hidden', was therefore more difficult to avoid than tomatoes and potatoes. There were no further reactions through the rest of the diet, so I told her to avoid potatoes and tomatoes and corn products.

In the next two to three months she continued to lose about three pounds per week and she remained totally free from depression. As I said earlier, all antidepressant medications had been stopped.

When I saw Jennifer again a few months later she was unrecognisable. Her weight had dropped to 8 stone 12 lb (124 lb or 56 kg) from the previous 13 stone 2 lb (184 lb or 83.5 kg). This represented a weight loss in total of 4 stone 4 lb (60 lb or 27 kg) without recourse to any form of calorie counting or quantity limitation. She ate as much as she liked of all foods other than the three foods identified as problematic for her. I saw her annually for the next six years and she remained the same, although she told me that she could now eat small amounts of corn occasionally without any adverse effects.

Case history 2: Judith H

Judith was 54 years old when she first talked to me about her weight gain. She was 5 feet 9 inches (1.75 metres) tall and weighed 11 stone 7 lb (161 lb or 73 kg), which she considered to be around 19 lb (8.5 kg) heavier than when she was in her twenties.

She had weighed this much for several years despite attending a high-impact aerobics class four times a week, and undertaking an 11 to 13 kilometre hike once a week. The only symptom she experienced was a frequently runny nose, but this was related to an allergy to house dust mites. She had no symptoms at all that would suggest food sensitivity other than her weight problem.

She went on to the elimination diet, as described in chapter 5, and (unusually for her) did experience a mild headache in the afternoon of the second day. By day six she felt much more alert than usual and didn't fall asleep in the evening while watching television, as previously she would have done. Her weight meanwhile had dropped from 11 stone 7 lb (161 lb or 73 kg) to 11 stone 0 lb (154 lb or 70 kg) by day seven. She was delighted to have lost seven pounds (3 kg) in seven days.

On Stage 2 – re-introduction of foods – she had no reaction to any of the 21 foods tested, and she lost another five pounds in those 10 days.

On the second and third day of Stage 3 – re-introduction of grains – she tested shredded wheat. By the evening of the third day she had gained four pounds, but had no symptoms. She correctly regarded this as an obvious reaction, so she stopped eating wheat. She did not test any other food for two more days till her weight had returned to what it had been before she tested the wheat.

She carried on testing other foods and when she tried corn (maize) her weight increased by five pounds by the second day of testing. By the end of Stage 3, despite these two reactions she had lost a further three pounds.

Three weeks later she had lost a total of 19 lb. This was right back to her ideal target weight of 10 stone 9 lb (149 lb or 67.5 kg). At no time did she ever feel hungry.

She decided to take desensitising injections for her two food sensitivities (wheat and corn) because these foods are so hard to avoid. She was then able to eat these without any further weight gain. She could, as they say, have her cake and eat it!

To many people Judith wasn't particularly overweight to start with, but she still managed to lose 19 lb and regain her youthful weight by a fairly straightforward procedure. She would be typical of millions of people who could achieve this response without any calorie or portion control.

Case history 3: Peter T

Peter was a 50-year-old man when he originally saw me in January 2007. He had a history of obesity, severe idiopathic oedema (unexplained fluid retention), considerable fatigue and very severe hypertension (high blood pressure). Idiopathic oedema is a generalised swelling, particularly around the ankles, caused by fluid retention. In my whole medical career I had never seen anyone with such severe oedema, extending up to way above his knees and with considerable swelling also of his hands and face. His weight was 20 stone 9 lb (289 lb or 131 kg) and his height was 5 feet 8 inches (1.73 metres).

Originally, when he first sought medical help, his blood pressure had been 260/130 mm Hg, which is dangerously high (normal is anything between 90/60 and 130/80). On his first appointment with me his blood pressure was 140/100 mm Hg, with a pulse rate of 100 beats per minute (normal is 72). This was despite taking 24 tablets a day as follows:

Breakfast:	Lisinopril 20 mg	1 tablet
	Frusemide 40 mg	4 tablets
	Amiloride 5 mg	3 tablets
	Aspirin 5 mg	1 tablet
	Metalazone 75 mg	½ tablet
	Isosorbide mononitrate	1 tablet

Lunch:	Hydralazine	2 tablets
	Doxazosin	2 tablets
	Spironolactone	2 tablets

Dinner:	Lisinopril	1 tablet
	Frusemide 40 mg	4 tablets
	Isosorbide mononitrate	1 tablet
	Bisoprolol	1 tablet

Peter had been told that he would need to keep taking this cocktail of diuretics, anti-hypertensives and aspirin for the rest of his life. He had gained the impression that this was not expected to be very long.

Peter was a builder by trade, and had not been able to work for two years. He suffered, as I said earlier, from considerable fatigue and having slept all night he would need a further six hours' sleep during the day.

In my clinical practice I had observed that many, but not all, patients with blood-pressure problems had lost these when embarking on an elimination diet. In 1978 I had collaborated with Dr Ellen Grant of the Migraine Clinic, Charing Cross Hospital, in a study of 60 patients with severe migraine. This study was later published in the *Lancet*.[4a] We put all patients in the trial onto my elimination diet as described in chapter 5. In 85% of these 60 patients, food sensitivity was discovered which, when addressed, resulted in all 85% losing their migraines. Fifteen out of the 60 patients had high blood pressure before starting the study, and all of these 15 found that, when they avoided the foods identified, their blood pressure returned to normal.

I was confident that Peter had a food sensitivity problem as I hadn't previously seen a case of oedema that had been caused by anything other than congestive cardiac failure and/or advanced renal disease, and Peter was not suffering from either of these conditions. I decided to put him on my elimination diet, as described in chapter 5. He continued to take his daily 24 tablets.

On the first day of the diet he felt as he usually did, but on the second day his oedema reduced spectacularly; however, he still felt very tired and short-tempered. By the third day his joints were a little sore but the oedema had continued to decrease to such an extent that he stopped all his diuretic tablets. On the fourth day he felt very odd and faint, and when he took his blood pressure it had reduced to 80/40 mm Hg. Very sensibly he rang me, so I advised him to discontinue some of his anti-hypertensives immediately and gradually to discontinue the rest. His blood pressure remained completely normal (120/80) for the last three days of the diet.

When I saw him on the seventh day he had no oedema at all anywhere on his body. He had lost 11 lb (5 kg) weight in seven days, and his waist measurement had reduced from 46 inches (117 cm) to 42 inches (106.5 cm). In addition, he told me he had lost all his fatigue and had been catching up with all sorts of tasks that he had been putting off for months. To summarise his progress, he had in seven days lost:

- 11 lb (5 kg) in weight
- 4 inches from his waist
- all of his swelling
- all of his fatigue
- his high blood pressure (now returned to normal)
- his need for any medication.

What a result in seven days, and what a dramatic demonstration of the effect that food sensitivity can have on a human being.

I then started reintroducing, mostly low risk, foods back into his diet, one new food at each of his three meals a day, with a minimum of five hours separating each meal. After about one week he tried consuming cows' milk. Within two hours he noticed his oedema coming back and a mild increase in blood pressure. These symptoms regressed within 36 hours as he obviously discontinued the milk. By day 17 of the diet he had lost a total of 25 lb (11.5 kg).

When I had taken his initial history I had noted that he had eaten wheat in one form or another at 80% of his meals, so I felt that cereal grains were most likely to be his main problem. I was fairly certain that wheat was going to cause a major reaction, as it is the single most common food sensitivity of all in the UK. I suggested that he tried oats instead; however, two hours after eating oats his legs and face became swollen again and there were clicking noises in his knees. A few days later, within five hours of introducing corn, the oedema in his legs had returned and he had an upset stomach, but no increase in blood pressure.

After cheddar cheese his blood pressure rocketed, and of course this ties up with his earlier reaction to milk.

He then tried wheat and reacted 'big time' as he put it. His blood pressure was 120/70 mm Hg before trying the wheat, and increased to 160/90 after the first meal. His oedema and fatigue returned in a spectacular manner. Later he had similar reactions to rye and monosodium glutamate. On completion of the diet he had lost a total of 4 stone 7 lb (63 lb or 28.5 kg).

Usually I offer desensitisation treatment if a patient is suffering from several major food sensitivities. The technique is described in some detail in chapter 6. Briefly here, foods are skin tested with extracts in various concentrations, between the surface layers of the skin. Usually doing this produces a small bubble (wheal) measuring approx 7 mm in diameter. If the patient is sensitive to that particular food the wheal will grow in size within 10 minutes, and quite often will cause the patient to experience slight symptoms. In Peter's case, when the wheat extract was given he had a wheal which increased in diameter from 7 mm to 12 mm after 10 minutes. His ankles and face started to swell and his blood pressure increased. He was then given the next strength of extract down and the wheal this produced also increased. The third strength down showed no wheal growth in size and the symptoms disappeared, so this was Peter's 'desensitising level' for wheat. His neutralising levels for other foods were also found.

In patients with multiple food sensitivities, like Peter, a cocktail of extracts of the neutralising concentration of each food is prepared, which the patient self-administers on alternate days. This enabled Peter to continue eating the foods he knew he was sensitive to.

Case history 4: Jennifer T

Jennifer T was 29 years old when she first attended my clinic. She had been around 16 years old when she first noticed having some headaches, but by the time she was 20 her migraines had started in earnest about once a month. Soon after she started taking the contraceptive pill the migraines had become more frequent and severe. Having tried three separate brands she reluctantly gave up the pill and the migraines improved somewhat. When she was 25 she married and by this time her headaches had worsened and she was also experiencing bouts of depression and general fatigue. She had had her first child at 27 and had developed post natal depression, but this had responded to one month's treatment with anti-depressants. However, her fatigue and migraines had become progressively worse, so her GP had tried various anti-depressants, tranquilisers and migraine preventive drugs. These treatments had only had marginal benefits. Over these few years her figure, that she had been so proud of, had increased from 9 stone to over 11 stone (her height was 5 feet 6 inches (1.68 metres)).

Discussing her worsening problems with her excellent GP, he had mentioned that he had read details of several clinical trials performed at London Teaching Hospitals which had convincingly demonstrated that most migraines were caused by everyday foodstuffs (85% of adults in several studies and 93% of children in one study). She told her GP she had already tried omitting cheese, chocolate, citrus fruits and red wine – all to no avail. He explained that commonly eaten foods such as wheat, eggs, yeast and various sugars seemed to be the more likely foods causing the problem. The foods involved vary enormously between individual patients, so he referred her to my clinic.

Having taken a history from her I told her that her experience of increasing weight, migraine and fatigue was extremely suggestive of food sensitivity as her GP had rightly suspected. I put her on my standard elimination diet as with the other patients I've described. She was warned that when she started this diet she would suffer a withdrawal reaction if her problems were indeed food sensitivity.

When she came to see me on the seventh day of the diet she ruefully confirmed that she had indeed had a severe migraine starting at lunchtime on the first day of the diet, being particularly intense in the evening of that day and all through the second day. The headache decreased in intensity on days three and four. The fatigue was also very bad on days two and three so she spent the second day of the diet in bed. After day four there was a noticeable improvement in her fatigue, but to her surprise she found that her muscles, particularly her thighs, buttocks and lower back ached as if she had flu. These symptoms are termed 'withdrawal myalgia' by doctors familiar with food sensitivity. These aches disappeared late on day five.

When she saw me on day seven, her eyes were sparkling and she could hardly contain her enthusiasm for the changes that had occurred in her health. She had lost 7 lb (3 kg) in the six days of the diet and in the last 48 hours she had lost the puffiness in her face and all traces of her fatigue. In addition, her mind felt clearer than it had done for years. I told her she had had a classic withdrawal reaction and that food sensitivity was certainly the root cause of her problems, including the weight gain.

As with the other patients, she then gradually reintroduced one food at a time. She reacted adversely to wheat, corn, oats, rye and malt, but no other foods were incriminated. The reactions to these foods varied slightly, but basically consisted of recurrences of all her symptoms and an increase in weight. Despite these reactions, in less than two months her weight had decreased back to 9 stone by simply avoiding these foods.

As these foods are difficult to avoid permanently I offered her specific desensitisation as described in the last two patients (see also chapter 6 for more detail). She continued with the desensitising treatment for two years and managed to keep her weight at around 9 stone and had no trace of the headaches, fatigue or depression she once had. I told her that after two years' treatment she could probably discontinue it while still eating the offending foods providing she didn't eat them in large quantities or daily. If she did eat the problem foods again in large quantities she would be likely to re-sensitise herself.

Case history 5: Amanda B

Amanda B was 33 years old when she first came to see me in 1992. She was a restaurant owner from Dorset. She was 5 foot 4 inches (1.63 metres) tall, and when I first saw her weighed 10 stone (140 lb or 63.5 kg). This does not seem too bad except that she had a very slight frame and delicate bone structure. Her normal weight had previously been 7 stone 7 lb (105 lb or 47.5 kg).

She told me that for over two years she had suffered from a very wide range of symptoms which included severe fatigue and pronounced weight variations, which could amount to 5–6 lb (2.25–2.75 kg) within 24 hours. There were also a lot of abdominal symptoms, including stomach pain, a hard bloated abdomen and constipation alternating with diarrhoea.

Also mentioned on the original questionnaire she completed for me were dehydration, dizziness, occasional palpitations, swelling of her ankles, cravings for sweet foods, feeling particularly bad first thing in the morning and even worse if she missed a meal. If she drank alcohol her back would become red and itchy.

Interestingly, most of her symptoms had started a few months after a bad attack of shingles and had become worse after glandular fever. Viral infections like glandular fever often seem to push people into food sensitivity problems.

When you read chapter 4 you will see that, like many people, she was an absolutely classic case of someone suffering from food sensitivities. Many physicians, however, would consider her problems to be psychosomatic due to the large number of symptoms present.

She went on to my elimination diet and stopped smoking her 20 cigarettes a day. By the evening of the first day she had a severe headache and the next four days were characterised by fatigue, depression, irritability and other problems. In other words, she experienced classic withdrawal symptoms. On day six of the diet, she felt a great deal better and by day seven all her abdominal symptoms had gone. She felt clear headed with no fatigue at all.

When I saw her at the end of Stage 2 (re-introduction of some foods) 10 days later she had in total lost 14 lb (6.5 kg) in weight and had reacted adversely to chicken, turkey, potatoes and broad beans. At the end of Stage 3 (re-introduction of grains) two weeks later she had reacted to wheat, corn, cows' milk and butter. She summarised her situation by announcing that she had lost 2 stone in weight (28 lb or 13 kg) and 27 symptoms in four and a half weeks. She opted for desensitisation to the foods to which she had reacted. The treatment worked well for most foods other than wheat, which she elected to avoid.

She also had some symptoms of the yeast syndrome described in chapter 7, which I treated with nystatin. A few months later when I saw her again she weighed 7 stone 7 lb (105 lb or 47.5 kg) which she considered to be the ideal weight for her slender frame. Thus she had lost a total of 2 stone 7 lb (35 lb or 16 kg) and all her symptoms.

She had a friend who was a journalist so her story became splashed all over the health pages of the *Daily Mail*.

Conclusion

There is one main point, in particular, that I would like to empha-sise about my elimination diet. At no stage throughout the proce-dure do I suggest any form of calorie or quantity restriction. You are able to eat as much of the allowed foods as you like. I have seen patients weighing over 20 stone losing 1.75 stone in seven days despite eating very large portions of food.

Some people may become worried about losing this amount of weight in such a short period of time. I would also be worried if the weight loss was a result of extreme calorie restriction, but in these cases all that is happening is that specific sensitive foods have been removed and this enables the body to regain its ability to normalise weight. I will say more about the body's mechanism for normalising weight in chapter 4.

Many of my patients had been calorie counting for years and had been restricting their intake to as little as 800–1000 calories per day before treatment. In contrast, on the elimination diet (see chapter 5) many have estimated that their calorie intake has been 2000–3000 calories each day.

A recurring theme is, 'How did I manage to lose such a large amount of weight in such a short time when I was eating so much?' The answer is simple. The root cause of the problem had been removed.

Around 75% of people with weight problems who complete my elimination diet achieve a major weight loss. They should need no further treatment, as long as they avoid the foods identi-fied as causing the problems. If, however, you do not reach your ideal weight, it may be because there are other complicating factors such as:

- the yeast syndrome (see chapter 7);
- problems with refined carbohydrates (see chapter 10);
- hypothyroidism (low production of thyroid hormones) (see chapter 8).

All but one of the five patients I have described had many other symptoms, and in fact, most people who are significantly overweight do have other problems such as headaches, migraine, fatigue, irritable bowel syndrome, joint pains and many more. These normally disappear on the diet as well as the weight. There are, however, some people who are overweight with no concurrent symptoms, such as Judith H, and these people can also have an excellent response to the approach described here. When such people introduce new foods into their diet they need to monitor their weight with an accurate set of scales, as described in the chapter on the elimination diet, as there will be no other indicators of a reaction.

I nearly always start any investigation of weight problems with my elimination diet, as specific food sensitivities can confuse other strategies such as low-carbohydrate diets (like the Atkins diet). The second and fourth patients described in this chapter would have done very well initially on any low-carbohydrate diet. You may recall that Judith just reacted adversely to wheat and corn, and Jennifer reacted to wheat, corn, rye and barley, but nothing else. None of these are allowed on the initial two- week induction phase of, for example, the Atkins diet. They would have suffered the same withdrawal symptoms that they encountered on my elimination diet and attained the same loss of weight and symptoms at the end of Stage 1. They would have then gone through the subsequent phases of the Atkins diet, and would have continued to progress. Eventually after several months, they would have re-introduced cereal grains. By this time they might have developed a mild degree of tolerance to the offending foods as they had avoided them for some time. When they first restarted eating them there would therefore have been no obvious reaction; however, this would not have continued and gradually the symptoms and weight would have returned. By this time they would have had no idea why a diet that seemed to be working so well had gone completely wrong and they would be back at square one. I have had to deal with this sequence of events frequently.

Conversely, I have seen a number of patients who have not responded well to diets such as Atkins because they are sensitive to eggs or cream, which are both very common food sensitivities and are allowed on all phases of low-carbohydrate diets. To be fair to Dr Atkins, he does recognise that food sensitivity and the yeast syndrome can both confuse the results of his dietary regime, and he devotes a whole chapter to each of these phenomena in his book. However, I do not agree with him on two very important points :

- My experience is that food intolerance is a more common problem than are high levels of insulin leading to insulin resistance;
- Dr Atkins recommends blood tests to identify food intolerances and I do not use them as I have found them to be hopelessly inaccurate.

Chapter 4

Understanding food sensitivity as a cause of weight problems

I will start this chapter with a statement that I have confirmed by successfully treating several thousand overweight patients in the course of over 30 years of clinical practice. I know it to be true for the UK, but am sure it also applies to many other countries.

Food sensitivities that are specific to each person are the single most common cause of weight problems.

Over 70% of people who are overweight, just slightly right through to those suffering from clinical obesity, will respond quite spectacularly to my elimination diet as described in the next chapter. If you have been frustrated for years with low-calorie or low-fat diets, you can lose considerable weight within seven days on my programme, and continue to lose weight as other foods are slowly restored to your diet.

You may have inadvertently observed this dramatic weight loss by going on a diet, commonly known as a 'fad' diet, that consists of only a few specific foods. The same thing quite often occurs if you go to one of the many health farms that offer a very restricted diet. If you find you lose lots of weight on one of the fad few-food diets, the weight loss achieved is more likely to be the result of avoiding certain specific foods, rather than of benefiting from the effects of the foods you are eating, or any consequent calorie restriction. This is essentially the same as what happens on my elimination diet. However, my approach involves taking the logical next step, which is to introduce common foods back into your diet, one at a time, to identify which are responsible for the problem in the first place.

My great awakening

As described in chapter 3, on 25 April 1976, I put Jennifer C on an elimination diet. The diet I put her on was far more restricted than the modern version I recommend in chapter 5. In seven days on this diet she lost all trace of her depression and 11 lb (5 kg) in weight. In the next few months she lost a total of 4 stone 4 lb (60 lb or 27 kg). She reacted to only three foods – tomatoes, potatoes and corn (but not wheat). On each reaction there was a recurrence of depression and a huge jump in weight, both of which disappeared within three days of discontinuing the offending food.

I was completely blown away by this turn of events and could hardly stop talking about it with anyone who would deign to listen. Was Jennifer a one-off fluke or was she typical of millions of people? Within three weeks of Jennifer's spectacular response to this diet I had put four other patients on the same programme, all of whom were substantially overweight and in addition had other symptoms. Amazingly, these next four patients all responded similarly, with impressive weight loss along with loss of other symptoms.

It wasn't until the ninth patient that this approach did not appear to work. (As I later came to realise, there are a number of causes of weight gain – which are often interconnected.) Already it was obvious to me that weight problems along with other medical conditions were frequently (about 80-85%) caused by food sensitivity. In the 31 years that followed I successfully treated thousands of patients with elimination diets. Over this period, with increasing experience I refined and adapted the diet until today I have defined the most effective choice of foods to identify problems while making life easier for those following it.

By 1982, I had become aware of other fundamental causes of weight problems and these are the subjects of later chapters in this book. I soon realised that I and my colleagues were moving towards a comprehensive view of what actually caused a great many health problems and chronic illnesses. Individual food sensitivity plays a very large part in that field.

A brief history of food sensitivity

The idea that foods can produce abnormal reactions has a long history and used to be the subject of considerable medical interest. The aphorism 'one man's meat is another man's poison' has been attributed to Lucretius, who lived about 100 years BC. For many centuries, dietary manipulations were one of the main areas of medical endeavour, but as interest in pharmacology grew in the last century, this concept were relegated to the backwaters of medicine. It has recently been demonstrated that this was a considerable oversight.

As long ago as 1905, Dr Francis Hare wrote an impressive two-volume book entitled *The Food Factor in Disease*. In it he outlined how he had successfully treated many patients with a wide variety of conditions by varying their diets. Later, in 1957, Dr Richard Mackarness wrote a best-seller called *Eat Fat and Grow Slim*. As you might imagine, this described a low-carbohydrate diet similar to the Atkins diet. This book sold over a million copies in the UK alone, which was quite an achievement for a non-fiction title at that time. While visiting the US to promote his book he met Dr Theron Randolph (see page 45), who introduced him to the concept of food sensitivity. Dr Mackarness was so impressed he then became more interested in food sensitivity than in low-carbohydrate diets. In 1976 he went on to write another book called *Not All in the Mind*, which was all about food sensitivity. I will say more about his work later in this chapter.

I was one of the first four doctors in the UK to become interested in this subject as a result of reading his book. I then went to the States to study the subject further, as there were several hundred physicians practising this type of medicine there.

There is no subject in medicine that has produced more confusion between doctors, or (even more so) between doctors and patients.

What are 'allergy', 'intolerance' and 'sensitivity'?

A lot of misunderstanding revolves around the definitions of 'food allergy', 'food intolerance' and 'food sensitivity'. These misunderstandings have occurred because over the years, since 1906 when the term 'allergy' was first used, the definition of 'food allergy' has changed in the minds of some doctors, but not in others. In 1906 an Austrian physician working in Vienna called Baron Clement Von Pirquet coined the term 'allergy', deriving it from two Greek words which together meant 'altered reactivity'. In other words, the term 'allergy' described a response to a substance which affected one individual, but not another.

At that moment in time (1906), nothing could be simpler. 'Food allergy' meant any individual reaction to a food, and therefore contrasted with 'toxicity', which adversely affects everyone, though usually to varying degrees. Thus everyone is killed by a large dose of hydrogen cyanide, but only some people react adversely to milk.

Then in 1925, the science of immunology was born, and it was discovered that certain types of allergy (that is, certain altered reactions) could be explained by the 'antigen-antibody hypothesis'. This hypothesis proposed that these reactions were the result of certain white blood cells, called 'mast cells' and 'basophils', being excessively activated by a type of antibody called immunoglobulin E (IgE). This type of reaction – called a 'type 1' reaction – rapidly results in an inflammatory response which can range from uncomfortable (hives, runny nose, eczema) to dangerous (asthma attack, or even anaphylactic shock – a major collapse often accompanied by significantly reduced blood pressure). Such reactions could be accurately measured in the laboratory and did not depend on the involvement of such unpredictable factors as actual patients.

Since that time it has come to be universally agreed that a food allergy is an immediate 'type 1' reaction to a food. It usually occurs in response to occasionally eaten, exotic foods, and generally the patient is more than aware of the problem as it happens almost immediately and is very obvious. This type of adverse reaction can be easily demonstrated by a blood test called the RAST test (the 'radioallergosorbent test'), which measures the levels of IgE antibodies in the blood in response to a specific substance, such as a food protein or an inhaled allergen (allergy inducing substance) such as pollens, dust, dust mites or moulds.

The term 'food intolerance' is frequently used for all adverse reactions to food which have not been shown to be IgE mediated. In the case of weight problems, virtually no foods that are implicated have been shown to be causing IgE-mediated responses. Of course, there are other ways in which human beings can react adversely to foods that are definitely not allergic responses by any stretch of the imagination. These include:

- **Enzyme deficiencies** – for example, deficiencies in the enzyme lactase, whose function is to digest the milk sugar called lactose. In this instance lactose is not digested properly and leads to lactose intolerance.
- **Toxicity** – certain foods can contain toxins - for example, the mould toxins that can be found in grain stored in damp conditions. These toxins (microtoxins) can produce symptoms in human beings.
- **The yeast syndrome (*Candida*)** – adverse reactions can, for example, be observed in response to eating sugar, and

this is probably because the sugar feeds the various yeasts that are involved in the problem (see chapter 7); alternatively, it may be a genuine reaction to yeasts in the gut.

The term **food sensitivity** is a sort of umbrella term which covers both food allergy and food intolerance. I have elected to use this term throughout the rest of this book because this dispenses with arguments about the precise mechanism involved. It makes no practical difference to the outcome for the individual person even if the academics find it fascinating.

What causes food sensitivity?

The short answer to this question is officially, 'We don't know.' The generally accepted view, however, from doctors working in this field is that food sensitivities arise from a monotonous, repetitive diet of foods that are relatively new to the human race, and often start in response to specific triggers. We have eaten meat, berries and nuts (but not peanuts) for two million years and are well adapted in general to these foods. We have eaten grain for only several thousand years, and milk, eggs and yeast for only a few thousand. These 'newer' foods are what might be described as the building blocks of the western diet and we eat them very often. Sensitivities to them may develop in response to a number of factors – for example, a bad viral infection, such as flu, shingles or glandular fever, may set them off.

As a result of treating countless patients with multiple food sensitivities combined with problems arising from the overgrowth of naturally occurring yeasts in the gut (see chapter 7) I think I know what is often at least partially to blame, as treating the yeast problem very often stabilises the food sensitivity problem, suggesting there is a relationship between the two. Yeast overgrowth, as described in much greater detail in chapter 7, may lead to the lining of the gut becoming excessively permeable; food that has been only partially digested can leak through such a 'leaky gut' and if the individual is not well adapted to those foods but eats them very frequently, s/he can easily sensitise him/herself to them.

Wouldn't I be aware if I had a food sensitivity?

The reason why almost everyone is totally unaware that they may have a food sensitivity is a phenomenon called '**masking**'. This concept is perhaps the single most important fact to grasp about food sensitivity. Most people are familiar with and understand the idea that someone can consume an occasionally eaten food and feel ill afterwards. Because of this, the public concept of food sensitivity has mostly been related to occasionally eaten and exotic foods. Many physicians also take this simplistic view of food sensitivity.

The concept of masked food sensitivity was originally identified by Dr Herbert Rinkel,[5] a well-known allergist practising in Oklahoma City. Dr Rinkel was renowned for being an extremely acute observer of various cause-and-effect relationships. After he qualified in medicine, he developed a severe nasal allergy called allergic rhinitis, which is a condition characterised by severe persistent nasal discharge. His medical colleagues skin-tested him for all the well-known inhalant allergies and these tests proved negative.

Dr Rinkel was familiar with a previous doctor's work on food sensitivity and suspected he might have such a problem himself. When he had been a medical student, like many of his colleagues he had been fairly poor. Grants are not common in the USA and, generally speaking, medical students going through college there have to support themselves or be supported by their parents. Rinkel's father, who was an egg farmer, had supported his son during his medical studentship by sending him a gross of eggs (144) each week, and this was the main source of protein for Rinkel and his family. This high comsumption of eggs continued after he qualified and he therefore suspected eggs as a cause of his problem. One afternoon, in an attempt to produce an adverse reaction, he consumed a particularly large quantity, but to his surprise his nasal symptoms that afternoon were, if anything, rather improved. Some months later he did the opposite; he abstained from eggs for about five days and then discovered that his nasal discharge improved considerably. After five days he inadvertently consumed some angel cake (which, of course, contained egg) at a birthday party. He suddenly collapsed with severe fatigue and his rhinitis returned in dramatic fashion.

Dr Rinkel suspected as a result of this experience that he might well have stumbled on something fundamental regarding the basic nature of food sensitivity. He thus repeated the experiment by re-establishing his consumption of eggs, omitting them again for five days and again repeating the egg ingestion, which caused a recurrence of the symptoms of fatigue and nasal discharge. He next extended his observations to a number of his patients and found a similar phenomenon occurring with a wide variety of different foods and with a wide variety of medical conditions. His observations were first published in 1944, when masking was defined in the following way:

- If a person ingests a particular food most days he or she may become sensitive to it and yet not suspect this as a cause of his/her symptoms.
- It is usual to feel better after a meal containing a food to which you have become sensitive than before the meal. In this case the feelings tend to **mask** the symptoms of the sensitivity. This is similar to someone who is addicted to cigarettes feeling a lot better after they have had one.

Dr Rinkel could not explain his observations.

Since Dr Rinkel's original work, cases of masked food sensitivity have been reported in millions of patients. Masked food sensitivity represents an interesting model of addictive behaviour and is, in my opinion, the major basic mechanism behind the cravings for such apparently diverse items as coffee, tea, milk, sugar, wheat, alcoholic beverages and tobacco. This concept can be represented graphically, as shown in Figure 4.1.

Figure. 4.1: Masked food sensitivity

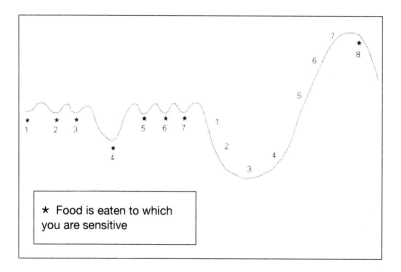

This graph illustrates the results of eating or not eating a masking food in someone with a single food sensitivity. Each star represents the eating of the food to which the person is sensitive. As can be seen, after the first meal the person's symptoms briefly improve and then start to get worse, but the second meal stops the deterioration. This is followed by another short period of improvement and then another decline. A similar response is experienced after the third time of eating. However, the fourth time of eating the sensitive food is delayed; this means the person's response occurs when s/he is further down the withdrawal curve and is thus feeling worse. Following this fourth ingestion, the person's condition returns to normal as the food is then eaten regularly (stars 5, 6 and 7).

In this example, after the seventh time of eating, the person has been told to avoid the offending food, and then exhibits the classic withdrawal phenomenon, characterised by a considerable deterioration in symptoms, usually by the evening of the first day. These symptoms may be headache or fatigue. The second and third days without the problem food tend to be quite severe, but they are followed by a slow improvement until the sixth day. By the sixth day most people are symptom free if under 35 years old. In those who are older, the symptoms may take another day or so to clear.

It is extremely gratifying to see someone with severe symptoms, clear of those for the first time for several years on the sixth or seventh day of this withdrawal period. Eating the food after the seventh day represents a deliberate re-presentation of the suspect food and this produces the hyper-acute response illustrated by Rinkel's experience – symptoms return quickly and quite dramatically on such occasions.

Figure 4.1 demonstrates how complicated the relationship is between one commonly eaten food and the symptomatology that it creates. Imagine, therefore, if a person has sensitivities to wheat, milk, corn and yeast; there will be a different curve of symptomatology for each food depending on the frequency at which it is eaten. Any relationship between food and symptoms will, in these circumstances, become far from obvious. I emphasise this point because many physicians believe that if food sensitivity is present, it will be obvious to all concerned. It is partly this simplistic view of the subject which has led to its neglect.

Individuals whose weight problems are related to food sensitivity usually see some weight loss by the third day of the elimination diet, and substantial weight loss by the seventh day. This usually amounts to about 5+ lb (2.5 kg) in a moderately overweight person, and occasionally up to 20 lb (9 kg) in a patient weighing around 24 stones (336 lb or 153 kg).

As I have already said, the concept of masking is the single most important factor to grasp about the inter-relationship between food and weight problems. It explains why so many overweight patients feel so bad in the morning. When they wake up they will have not had a masking dose of the problem food for around 12 hours.

The development of food sensitivity and its consequences

A common sequence of events that occurs initially in someone developing, say, a milk sensitivity early in life goes as follows: at first it may lead to a rash or runny nose; later, if the cause of these symptoms is not identified (as is usually the case) the symptoms may become more generalised and include the gaining of weight. Since the consumption of milk continues on a daily basis the symptoms blur from one day to another and the role of milk becomes totally hidden.

In fact the person will probably become a 'milk-oholic', learning subconsciously that if they maintain their intake of milk in any form they will feel less ill than if they avoid it. Of course they will continue steadily to gain weight.

I met Dr Theron Randolph in 1978 and later spent two weeks working with him. He had developed the concept of an 'addiction pyramid'. In this concept a person may, as a child, become intolerant/addicted to foodstuffs, particularly grains, sugar, milk or eggs. This may eventually lead to a number of different symptoms such as migraine, hyperactivity, fatigue, or bowel problems. Such a child may then go on in his/her teens to become intolerant/addicted to other things such as coffee and a wide variety of other foods, even including alcohol in some cases. Alcoholic drinks are, after all, just mixtures of foods like yeast, grapes, sugars and grains. Dr Randolph coined the phrase 'reactions to alcoholic drinks represent food sensitivity in a jet propelled vehicle' as they are absorbed so rapidly. This is, of course, an extreme example; most people experience a much milder form of the problem.

Fixed and cyclic food sensitivities

Food sensitivities can be divided into fixed food sensitivities and cyclic food sensitivities. A fixed food sensitivity is one which has probably been present since birth and will never go away. In other words, the individual may eat the food extremely rarely but will react adversely every time. He or she may avoid the food for 20 years and then still react strongly to it. These fixed food sensitivities are comparatively rare and certainly account for less than 5 % of all food sensitivities. They are nearly always the classic IgE-mediated type allergic reactions as described earlier.

A food sensitivity which disappears within two years of complete avoidance of the food will generally be regarded as cyclic food sensitivity. In cyclic food sensitivity, the degree of reaction is related to how often it is eaten. One method of treatment, other than the 'desensitisation' that is discussed in chapter 6, is to avoid the food for a period of time, during which tolerance can develop. This time usually varies between two and eight months, but by definition can extend for up to two years. Usually the stronger the reaction that the food produces, the longer it takes for a tolerance to develop. Tolerance can also, in exceptional circumstances, develop within four or five weeks and this is a possible source of problems in the elimination diet, which may extend over a period of six or seven weeks.

Tolerance is, however, a fragile flower and can usually be maintained only if you eat the food to which you were sensitive no more frequently than once a week. If the food is consumed more frequently than that, you nearly always start to react to it again. It is, of course, vital to understand this concept. I have seen patients who have identified specific food sensitivities on an exclusion diet and then some months later have eaten the food again by mistake but, having suffered no reaction, conclude that their original observation was erroneous. Unless fore-warned, they may then start to eat the food on a frequent basis, rapidly destroy their tolerance of it, and then start to react to it once more.

What are the most common foods that I might be sensitive to?

During more than 30 years of experience with thousands of patients I have identified the 20 foods most likely to produce a reaction. Over this period of time there have also been numerous clinical studies that have arrived at very similar findings. I have listed the foods in order of frequency, starting with the most common:

1. wheat
2. corn (maize)
3. milk and products made from milk
4. eggs
5. yeast (used in many products such as bread, vinegar and alcohol)
6. cane sugar
7. coffee
8. oats
9. rye
10. barley (malt)
11. beet sugar
12. tea
13. potatoes
14. soy (used frequently in processed foods)
15. lemons
16. cocoa beans (chocolate)
17. oranges
18. beef
19. pork
20. onions

These foods are, of course, the most commonly eaten in the UK. There are slight variations between different western countries, so for example, in the USA corn is the most commonly eaten grain, hence corn is the commonest cause of sensitivity.

The position of each food on the list varies a little for different medical conditions. In migraine, for example, although wheat is still the most common, oranges would be at around position three or four. Only around 2% of migraine sufferers react only to cheese, chocolate, citrus fruits and red wine, contrary to popular belief. You will probably find that you react only to a handful of foods, and if you are lucky, just one or two. Occasionally someone will react to something obscure like pineapple or melon.

I would like to reassure you that all the foods in my elimination diet do not feature in the list of the top 60 foods to which you are likely to react.

How weight is regulated normally and what happens when it goes wrong

Enter the 'lipostat' (not to be confused with the medicine, Lipostat – a statin). In 1970 Gordon Kennedy,[6] at Cambridge University UK, described what he called the 'lipostat theory of body weight control'. This proposes a feedback mechanism whereby an area in the part of the brain called the hypothalamus responds to signals that stored body fat has increased, prompting the individual to be more active and less hungry.

When this mechanism is working well your body weight remains surprisingly constant, despite quite widely varying calorie consumption from day to day. The mechanism defends us against calorie deprivation or calorie over consumption. However, the adverse reaction caused by individual foods to which you are sensitive, if eaten daily, causes the lipostat to be permanently set at the wrong level. As the foods implicated usually are those that you do eat every day, or almost every day, this problem remains constant, as does the adverse effect on your weight. Thus identifying the fundamental causes of your weight problem is the only successful way forward. What is remarkable in people with major weight problems caused by food sensitivity is that they notice wide variations in their weight within each 24 hours, so much so that they often have one set of clothes which they wear in the morning, and another set for the evenings.

If your lipostat is working how you would like it to, life becomes easier. If, however, it is not, thanks to certain food sensitivities, efforts to try and treat weight problems with just calorie or fat reduction are doomed. If you eat less your lipostat will tell your body it needs to take in more food and be less active. The lipostat is a very powerful mechanism; if you try to override it, in the long term it will win. Sort out what is upsetting it – for example, food sensitivity, yeast toxins or low thyroid output – and you will win.

The work of Dr Richard Mackarness

As I have already mentioned earlier in this chapter, in the late 1950s, a British doctor, Richard Mackarness, stumbled upon the concept of food allergy and sensitivity. He had noted that people who lived in primitive circumstances eating primitive foods rarely became obese, and he thought that obesity might result from foods such as cereals and sugars, products which had only comparatively recently been incorporated into the human diet. Whereas fruits, vegetables, meats and fish had been consumed for several million years, cereals had been consumed for only about 10,000, and sugar for approximately 300. In England, cereals have probably been consumed for only 2000 years. It is thus possible that mankind, particularly in this part of the world, has not had time to adapt to these comparatively new foods. In his book *Eat Fat and Grow Slim*, against the prevailing medical wisdom of the day, he advocated a diet avoiding cereals and sugars, but allowing as much fat, protein, vegetables and other carbohydrates as the individual required.

Many people found this diet very helpful and the book sold in enormous quantity in the UK. As a result, his publishers asked him to do a lecture tour of the USA to promote the launch of the book there. At one of these lectures he met a doctor who, having listened to his lecture, said to him, 'I am sure that you are right, but possibly for the wrong reasons. Many of your patients are probably sensitive to foods such as cereals and sugars. By telling them not to eat these foods, they are probably becoming better because they are avoiding the common food sensitivities.' It is, of course, likely that these foods are the most common causes of food sensitivities because mankind has not adapted well to them.

This doctor suggested that Dr Mackarness should meet his brother-in-law, Dr Theron Randolph, whose ideas I have already mentioned on page 45. Dr Mackarness responded to this idea with alacrity and became fascinated by the ideas that Dr Randolph was able to impart. When Dr Mackarness returned home he slowly incorporated these new ideas into his day-to-day practice, while tending to lose interest in low-carbohydrate diets. Having acquired a fair amount of experience in this field and having become entirely convinced by its validity, he then wrote *Not All in the Mind*, which was initially published in 1976. In 1980 he followed this success with *Chemical Victims*. With these two books he succeeded in opening up awareness of this approach.

Spreading the word

Although the medical profession as a whole was not interested in food and chemical sensitivity, a small group of doctors, of which I was one, had their curiosity aroused. In 1979, about 19 doctors formed the British Clinical Ecology Group. By January 1982 the number had swelled to over 100 and changed its name to The British Society for Allergy and Environmental Medicine.

When we joined the British Society for Nutrition Medicine, their name was incorporated into ours leading to the British Society for Allergy, Environmental and Nutrition Medicine. This was a bit of a mouthful and so finally the name changed to The British Society for Ecological Medicine.

Various clinical trials began to be published which linked food sensitivity with human illness. There are over 7500 published studies examining the role of food allergy and sensitivity in human health. They include papers on migraine, fatigue, irritable bowel syndrome, Crohn's disease, ulcerative colitis, rheumatoid arthritis, renal disease, cardiac disease, asthma, rhinitis and many other conditions. Most of them are described in detail in the major textbook *Food Allergy and Intolerance* edited by Professor Jonathan Brostoff and Dr Stephen Challacombe.

Tests for food sensitivity

1. Elimination diets

Elimination diets are undoubtedly the 'bench-mark' against which all the other methods of testing should be measured. When going through an elimination diet you see in real life what is happening. If you have weight problems, limiting your diet for seven days to a handful of safe foods (not the quantity of food eaten), as described in the chapter 5, will let you know where you stand if you experience a loss in weight. It is not a great sacrifice when a few days can change your whole future outlook from unmitigated pessimism to great optimism. The test also has the virtue that it is both simple and inexpensive. If reasonable weight loss is not achieved by seven (or eight in those over 35) days, then food sensitivity can be excluded.

The subsequent phase of reintroducing foods into your diet may be just as simple, but it is fair to say that in someone with a large number of sensitivities it can be very complicated.

2. Intradermal provocative skin-testing and neutralisation

This approach is a vast improvement on, and refinement of, standard skin prick-testing which has been used for many years in hospitals. There have been about 12 clinical trials which have established its validity and, used competently, it is a vital and extremely useful method of both diagnosis and treatment. About six clinics in the UK use the test extensively, and in the USA it is used currently by over 300 clinics. Without it we would not be able to help a large proportion of our more complicated patients. The test and concept are so important that I have devoted a whole chapter to the uses of this method (chapter 6).

3. Prick testing

This is a fairly useful test for inhalant allergies, but does not really help in the diagnosis of food sensitivity. It is this simple fact which has, in my opinion, held back until recently the development of interest in food sensitivity.

The test involves placing a single drop of allergen extract on the inner forearm. A lancet is introduced through the drop of extract on the skin at an acute angle and, having slightly penetrated the skin, is given a deliberate vertical lift before being removed. Responses to these tests are read after 10 to 20 minutes, and many of these tests can be performed within a few minutes of each other. The whole test is, therefore, both simple and quick to perform. Unhappily, it is not very effective because most patients with well-established food sensitivities will fail to react positively to it. To practitioners using the intradermal provocative neutralising test it has become apparent why prick tests are so useful for diagnosing inhalant allergies but useless for diagnosing food sensitivities – the inherent risks of the skin prick tests have resulted in them being done at such weak concentrations that they will generally miss food sensitivies, whose neutralising levels are usually rather higher than levels for inhaled allergens.

Unfortunately, because prick tests have been used for so long, many people, including physicians, place unwarranted credence on their results. I have known patients with genuine food sensitivities be informed categorically that their sensitivities do not exist, purely on the basis of this type of test. This can therefore do more harm than good. Dr Keith Eaton of Reading described a trial he carried out showing that the prick test is of no value in diagnosing food sensitivities. He showed that the reliability of the test was only 15% for foods. As he put it himself, 'One is better off tossing a coin to determine food sensitivities as this has a reliability of 50%.'

4. RAST test

'RAST' is short for 'radioallergosorbent test' and only measures IgE-mediated allergy (as already described), which is irrelevant in weight management. I have never known such an allergy to cause weight problems.

5. Other blood tests

There is a range of blood tests on the market which purport to be able to diagnose food sensitivity. If this were really true and the tests were accurate it would totally revolutionise medicine. Any doctor could then draw a blood sample, and send it to an appropriate laboratory. Unhappily, in my long experience, they are not reliable and the results in most cases bear little or no relationship to the true reality of the situation. I know of only one doctor from the Society of Ecological Medicine who uses them.

Professor W J Rea from Dallas, Texas is arguably the leading authority in the world on this subject. He told me that in his opinion there are at least six different mechanisms involved in food sensitivity and no one test could encompass all of these differing factors.

In 1995 when I was president of the British Society for Allergy, Environmental and Nutritional Medicine I was approached by a company that was just starting to promote a new blood test for food sensitivities. They asked me to endorse their product. I told them I was not known for my enthusiasm for blood tests based on my previous experience in this area. They assured me that their test was quite different. I told them that I would be delighted to give my endorsement if they could prove the accuracy of their test in patients where I already knew exactly what the answer should be. To my amazement they agreed to this, and to carry out the tests free of charge as they were not actually required by the patients involved. I sent blood samples from the next 12 patients who had successfully completed my elimination diet. They had lost all of their symptoms, and had found it easy to identify the 'offending' foods.

The first patient had rheumatoid arthritis and having lost all joint pains on the initial diet, then reacted subsequently to wheat, corn, oats, rye and malt. The laboratory informed me he had reacted to lamb, eggs, milk and potatoes. He was, however, eating all these foods without any problems. They had completely missed all the cereal grain reactions. None of the next 11 patients was correctly diagnosed. The best results were from three patients where the laboratory managed to pick up three of their five sensitivities; however, for each they also identified foods that were not a problem. Needless to say this laboratory did not get my endorsement. If I had my way I would make all laboratories be subjected to this type of evaluation before being able to advertise their services.

This is very much an all or nothing subject. Still eating two foods that are problematic won't lead to much improvement in weight management. If you have three drawing pins sticking through the sole of your shoe, removing two might be an improvement, but walking is still going to be painful!

Treatment for food sensitivities

The only effective specific treatment for individual food sensitivities is the 'intradermal provocative neutralisation' technique, involving tiny self-administered injections every other day. This is described in detail in chapter 6. It is offered by over 100 clinics in the USA, but is available in only a few in the UK (see appendix II).

Chapter summary

- In April 1976 I put a patient, who was four and a half stone overweight, on an elimination diet. She also had depression. In just seven days she lost 11 lb (5 kg) in weight, and her depression. She discovered that only three foods caused all of her problems and by the end of three months she had lost all four and a half stone of excess weight.
- In the next 31 years I saw thousands of other patients with similar responses, some with more, and some with less, weight to lose. After all that experience, I consider that around 75% of people will respond to my elimination diet by losing all or most of their excess weight.
- Most people never suspect that everyday foods (unfortunately often their favourites) are the root cause of all of their problems. This is a result of a phenomenon called 'masking', in which the repeated consumption of certain offending foods makes it impossible to identify which foods are causing weight gain. Only by going on a scientifically structured elimination diet is it possible to get to the root of the problem.
- The top five problem foods in the UK are wheat, corn,

dairy products, eggs and yeast. In the US the top food is corn.

- The only reliable test for food sensitivities other than going on an elimination diet is intradermal provocative skin-testing.
- The only truly effective method for dealing with a food sensitivity is either to avoid the food or to use the intradermal provocative neutralisation technique, offered by several clinics in the UK and many clinics in the USA (see appendix II).

Chapter 5

The elimination diet

An elimination diet is the most useful tool of all for sorting out the food sensitivities that can lead to weight problems. It is cheap and perfectly safe. As you might expect, most people find such a diet to be easy to follow and easy to assess. However, you must be aware at the outset that the whole process will take at least six weeks to complete and once started you cannot give yourself any 'days off', especially in the first two weeks.

People with weight problems fall into two categories: those who have no other problems at all, and those who do have other health problems. Typically these might be headaches, migraine, fatigue and bowel problems. In fact, it is very common for people who experience difficulty in keeping down their weight to have these kinds of symptoms as well.

During the first seven days of my elimination diet if you have no other symptoms at all, all you may notice is an impressive loss of weight. If you are one of the people who do experience other problems you may notice a worsening of these symptoms in the first three or four days of the diet followed by a marked improvement by day six or seven. This response is perfectly normal and will usually accompany a significant loss of weight. You may, by day seven, feel significantly brighter and more energetic than before you embarked on the diet. Previously you may well have blamed feelings of mild fatigue and low energy on other factors, such as growing older;

finding they improve can be a real unexpected bonus. It is further confirmation that you are on the right track.

On the seventh day you can start introducing more foods back into your diet, one each morning and one each evening. This is described in detail in the rest of this chapter.

The elimination diet

Stage 1

The elimination diet starts with a low-risk selection of foods. There are 42 foods which, in my 30+ years of experience, have a very low risk of causing reactions. They are listed in Table 5.1. These foods are used simply 'to keep the wolf from the door' while you avoid all the likely incriminating foods.

All of these foods can be cooked in any way providing you *use only water or olive oil or roast in own juices*. This initial diet lasts for only seven days.

Table 5.1 Foods that can be eaten at Stage 1

Meats (including liver or kidneys)	
Duck	Turkey
Lamb	Venison
Fish (fresh or plain frozen*)	
Cod	Trout
Haddock	Sea Bass
Mackerel	Sea Bream
Monkfish	Skate
Plaice	Swordfish
* not in batter, breadcrumbs, sauce or marinade of any kind, or tinned or smoked	

High carbohydrate vegetables	
Lentils	Sweet potatoes
Parsnips	Turnips
Swedes	
Vegetables	
Courgettes (zucchini)	Peas
Green beans	Spinach
Marrow	
Salad	
Avocado	Lettuce (any variety)
Celery	Olives (green or black)
Chinese bean sprouts	Water cress
Cucumber	
Fruit (fresh only)	
Apples	Persimmon (sharon fruit)
Peaches	Pineapple
Pears	Plums
Nuts (not roasted or salted)	
Cashews	Pistachio
Macadamia	

NB: If you regularly eat any of the foods listed at least three times a week, that food should be omitted from the diet and not added back in until the end of Stage 3. Olive oil can be an exception to this, even if you cook with it daily.

Any strict vegetarian who wishes to do this diet would, of course, have to omit the fish and meat. Any elimination diet is inevitably more difficult for vegetarians.

The only liquid which is allowed on the diet is one of the bottled mineral waters. It does not appear to matter whether the water is still or sparkling, and this can be left to your personal taste. Should you wish to liquidise the fruits with the spring water and make a fruit juice, this would be fine.

Pure sea salt can be used for flavouring the food.

There remains one further piece of advice which you should follow: A large dose of Epsom salts should be taken on the first morning of the elimination diet to evacuate foods consumed on the preceding days. Two teaspoons of Epsom salts are adequate for most adults. These should be dissolved in about ¼ pint (140 ml) of spring water. Do not be tempted to use other brands of laxatives as they may contain confusing ingredients.

I must emphasise that the foods listed above are the ONLY foods that you can eat on Stage 1 of this diet. There can, therefore, be no tea, no coffee, no bread, no milk, no sugar, no eggs – nothing that is not listed. It is also important to note that chewing gum is not allowed, as it often contains sugar, starch or artificial sweeteners, all of which may cause problems.

Quite often when people first look at this list the first words that escape their lips are: 'What am I going to have for breakfast?' Now breakfast for most people actually contains the foods that are most frequently known to cause problems. High on the list of problem foods are wheat, corn, milk and eggs. All of these are, I am afraid, banned for the time being. What you can eat with minimal preparation are fruits, nuts, salads (possibly with a little olive oil and salt) or cold meat from last night's roast. The main meal of the day can contain a large quantity of fish or meat with plenty of vegetables, finishing with some fruit.

Eating in restaurants or at social occasions is very difficult. I advise avoiding this definitely in the first week and ideally in the second week as well. If you know you have a big event coming up it is better to delay starting till it is over.

What to expect

The overriding concern in the latter part of the first week is to observe a large decrease in weight by day seven, with probable improvement in other symptoms if there are any. Obviously a person who is five stone overweight is liable to lose more weight in the first seven days than someone who is overweight by one stone.

Stage 2

The prime objective of Stage 2 is to expand your diet as quickly as possible. To that end you should select, especially in the first three or four days, foods which are unlikely to give adverse reactions (see next section). That should be followed by foods which are generally desirable, but have only a moderate risk of causing sensitivity. The order of introduction follows this rule which is important to stick to rigidly: introduce the safer foods earlier; in addition, separate the introduction of members of similar food families by four days to avoid confusion through cross-reactivity within specific food families.

Two new foods should be added each day, starting with one new food on the evening of day seven, after evaluating your progress earlier that day. One food should be tested in the morning at breakfast time and one in the evening, thus allowing at least nine hours between tests. This should be adequate time for any reaction to develop. Lunchtime is limited to those foods that were permitted on Stage 1 or which have already been passed as safe on Stage 2. It does not matter on any particular day which of the two foods is tested in the morning and which in the evening.

Stage 2 order of food reintroduction

Day 7	(evening) Broccoli
Day 8	Red/green/yellow/orange peppers
	Chicken
Day 9	Brown rice
	Bananas
Day 10	Tap water (to check you do not react to any of the chemicals in it)
	Black tea (whichever tea you normally consume, but without milk, lemon or sugar)

Day 11	Cows' milk (WHOLE milk)
	Grapes
Day 12	Onions
	Pork
Day 13	Ground coffee
	Lemon
Day 14	Eggs
	Melon
Day 15	Beef
	Yeast (bread-making yeast – 2 teaspoons – possibly mixed with banana if the banana test has been satisfactory)
Day 16	Butter
	Cabbage
Day 17	Potatoes
	Dry white wine (if no problems with yeast or grapes)

In the event of one of the foods being unavailable, fresh (not tinned) tuna or salmon can be substituted. It is important not to introduce any food before the day specified as foods in individual food groups have been specifically kept apart.

When testing a food, the most important thing to watch for is a sudden increase in weight. However, if headache, fatigue, or other symptoms occur, it is still sensible to regard this as a reaction and drop the food from your diet, at least for the time being. Symptoms most commonly occur within four or five hours, but 9 or 10 hours are recommended between tests to accommodate people who tend to react slowly.

Weight monitoring should be employed all through Stages 2 and 3. It is essential that a good quality digital weighing machine should be purchased and weight measurements made early morning (before breakfast) and early evening (before the evening meal).

Table 5.2 gives an example of someone who weighed 11 stone 5 lb (159 lb or 72 kg) before beginning Stage 1, and on the seventh day weighed 10 stone 11 lb (151 lb or 68.5 kg). This is a record of how her weight responded to each food added. Obviously you will probably not react to the same foods, but her experience will give you an idea of what to look out for and how to proceed.

Table 5.2 Case history: weight variation while introducing foods at Stage 2

Day	Weight (before breakfast) Stone lb	Food tested	Weight (before evening meal) Stone lb	Food tested
7	10.11	Usual Stage I foods	10.13	Broccoli
8	10.10	Red/green peppers	10.12	Chicken
9	10.09	Bananas	10.11	Brown rice
10	10.09	Tap water	10.11	Black tea
11	10.08	**Cows' milk**	**10.13**	**No food tested**
12	**10.10**	**No food tested**	**10.11**	**No food tested**
13	10.08	Grapes	10.10	Pork
14	10.07	Onion	10.09	Lemon
15	10.07	Ground coffee	10.09	Melon
16	10.06	Eggs	10.08	Beef
17	10.06	**Yeast**	**10.10**	**No food tested**
18	**10.08**	**No food tested**	**10.09**	**No food tested**
19	**10.07**	**No food tested**	10.08	Butter
20	10.06	Cabbage	10.08	Potatoes

You can see from this schedule that this person usually gained about two pounds as the day progressed which were then lost during the night. This was, of course, because she was eating during the day but not at night.

The 'before breakfast' weight reading usually decreased by about one pound every other day. If weight is lost or stable from one day to the next you can be sure that both new foods eaten for the first time on that day must be OK.

In this example you can see the 'before breakfast' and 'before evening meal' readings decreased every day until Day 12. On Day 11 cows' milk had been introduced after the normal 'before breakfast' reading. During that day, instead of gaining the usual two pounds there was a five-pound increase. Cows' milk was therefore very likely to be a food sensitivity in this case. When this happens, consuming cows' milk (or whatever the food is in your case) should cease and no new food should be tested until the reaction has worn off.

The slow downward drift in weight then continued until yeast was tried. This caused another temporary rise in weight. Thus, in this example, both cows' milk and yeast should, for the time being be removed from the diet. Yeast is tested at this stage in the programme because it is a common ingredient of many foods to be tested later. Both cows' milk and yeast should, at some time, be retested, but early on I think it is more important to find more 'good' foods, to expand your diet as quickly as possible.

If, in addition, any symptoms recur at the same time that weight increases, this definitely confirms that you have a sensitivity to that food.

Essential rules

I should like to emphasise that once you have found that a food does not cause any reaction it can then be eaten whenever you like from then onwards (but see the note about rye on page 69). However, the most important rule to obey is: NEVER RE-TEST A FOOD WITHIN FIVE DAYS OF THE ORIGINAL TEST. The only time an immediate reaction to a food occurs is when it has been omitted from the diet for a minimum of five days. If it is omitted for a shorter period than this, a reaction will occur, but it will be delayed and possibly not be associated with that food. Thus the three major rules of food testing are:

- Once you have found a food does not cause a reaction you can eat it whenever you like from then onwards.
- If in doubt about a food reaction, leave the food out of the diet.
- Never re-test a food in less than five days from the original test.

You must, therefore, restrict yourself to those foods already found to be safe until the weight gain and/or symptoms pass. This of course slows up the testing programme and all the timing of reintroducing foods on certain days will change. To speed up the clearing of a reaction, the following mixture is strongly recommended:

2 teaspoons of sodium bicarbonate

1 teaspoon of potassium bicarbonate

These two bicarbonates should be placed in ¼ pint (140 ml) of hot water and stirred until dissolved. The sodium bicarbonate is ordinary bicarbonate of soda, which is obtainable at any chemist or supermarket. The potassium bicarbonate can be quite difficult to obtain. However, your chemist should be able to get it from a wholesaler. The mixture is pretty revolting to take and most people prefer to swallow it in one gulp. It usually does two things:

- It gives you a bowel movement, and the food to which you are reacting tends to be eliminated from your intestines. Clearly, the faster this occurs the better.
- Food reactions are accompanied by a reactionary acidosis: all your body fluids become slightly more acid, and this indirectly causes many of the symptoms. A large dose of alkali corrects this situation to some extent.

This medication, therefore, acts in two separate and complementary ways. A single dose of the bicarbonate mixture will normally halve the reaction time. If you can face a further dose it can be taken four to six hours later to further help the reaction to subside. The time for you to restart testing is when the weight gain (and/or symptoms) from the preceding reaction have subsided.

Stage 3

You can now embark on Stage 3, which involves many foods with the potential to cause problems, including the cereals, which need special consideration in their testing. Cereals, especially wheat, are very slowly absorbed and most frequently take 36 hours to cause a reaction. I have even seen some patients take more than two days to react to wheat, and this, therefore, must be taken into account.

Day 18	Carrots
	Oranges
Day 19, 20 & 21	Wheat
	Test either as wholewheat spaghetti or pure shredded wheat. Shredded wheat is probably the best test, but it is difficult to consume if milk has not been found to be satisfactory on the last stage. The pure wheat should be eaten at all meals on these three days (plus any of the safe foods). The reaction to this foodstuff is not only slow to materialise, but if it occurs it is very slow to eradicate. I have seen some patients take four to five days before they feel well again.
Day 22	Wholemeal bread
	This should only be tested if both the wheat test and the yeast test have been satisfactory. Try wholemeal bread at each meal for this day.

Day 23   Instant coffee test
              Use Nescafe Gold Blend as this is another chemical
              test, predominantly for preserving chemicals. Cau-
              tion – many cheap coffees contain corn.
              Tomatoes

Day 24   Cane sugar
              This should be a Jamaican, Trinidadian or other West
              Indian demerara sugar. Muscovado is also suitable.
              Two teaspoons of cane sugar should be eaten three
              times a day for one full day.

Day 25   Mushrooms
              Peanuts
              The peanuts should be obtained loose from a health
              food shop. Do not use the packet varieties, which have
              additives.

Day 26   Beet sugar
              This is retailed under the name of Silver Spoon in
              the UK and marketed by the British Sugar Corpora-
              tion. Usually it is pure beet sugar, but sometimes, if
              the beet sugar crop has been inadequate in quantity,
              there can be a little cane sugar added to it. Reactions
              to cane sugar and beet sugar are quite separate, as
              they come from totally different plants Please note
              that Tate & Lyle sugar has both cane sugar and beet
              sugar in some products. Spend one day on testing
              beet sugar, taking two teaspoons at each meal.

Day 27 & 28   Corn
              This very commonly consumed food should be tested
              in two forms (1) corn on the cob, and (2) pure glucose
              powder. Glucose retailed in Britain is nearly always

made from corn, although most retail chemists are unaware of this. Start each meal with fresh or frozen corn on the cob (or loose, but not tinned in case of added sugar) and finish the meal with two teaspoons of glucose. Take both forms of corn at each meal for two full days. Some people appear to react more obviously to one form of corn and some to the other. Either way, the reaction is to corn. Reactions to corn are slow but usually not quite as slow as to wheat and I have not seen them starting more than 48 hours after commencing this test.

Day 29   Cheddar cheese (even if you are sensitive to milk)
Soya milk (pure and unsweetened)
Soy is very important. It is present in soya-bean oil (vegetable oils), soya-bean flour, etc. One way or another it is present in an extensive range of manufactured foods.

Day 30   Black pepper
Bacon (if pork is satisfactory)
When testing for bacon you are, in fact, testing for the nitrite and nitrate chemicals that have been used to make bacon. Check there is no sugar mentioned on the packet.

Day 31   Grapefruit
Chocolate
Chocolate contains wheat, corn and sugar. Do not test if you have found you are sensitive to any of these items.

Day 32 & 33   Rye
Use Ryvita (the original rye crispbread). Eat rye at every meal for two full days unless a reaction occurs

sooner. If you should react to rye and you have already reacted to wheat, I do not think it is worthwhile testing oats or malt later, as reactions to these will by now be a foregone conclusion. It is wise to eat rye a little cautiously if a wheat sensitivity has already been detected. Rye and wheat are very closely related in the botanical tables, and many people who are sensitive to wheat will soon sensitise themselves to rye if they eat a lot of it. Becoming sensitive to rye is the most common cause of confusion and dismay on the last part of my elimination diet.

Day 34   White bread (do not test if you are sensitive to wheat, yeast or corn – or soy if this is on the list of ingredients)
This is a test for chemicals, especially anti-staling agents, which are present in white bread retailed in the UK.

Day 35   Prawns or shrimps
Monosodium glutamate
This is a flavour enhancer used in many tinned foods, sauces, gravies, etc. It can be obtained in pure white crystalline form in many supermarkets (especially Chinese) and delicatessens. A little of the powder should be sprinkled like salt over some meat, or almost any other foodstuff you prefer.

Day 36   Aspartame
Test in the form of the artificial sweetener called NutraSweet.
Raisins (do not test if sensitive to grapes)
Here you are testing the chemicals used that are also in currants, sultanas and other dried fruits.

Day 37 & 38   Oats
Ideally eat porridge oats at every meal for two days or until a reaction occurs.

Day 39   Cauliflower
Any other fresh fruit of your choice.

Day 40   Malt
Test for one full day. Take two teaspoons of malt extract at every meal. This must be five days after a positive reaction to testing oats, in which case it must be left to day 44. You can use pearl barley in homemade soups as well. This is another 'hidden' ingredient common in some foods e.g. beer, vinegar.

End of Stage 3 assessment

If you have tried all the foods at each stage, you will have in effect assessed 84, which account for 95 % of what most people eat. Fruits such as cherries, raspberries, gooseberries and blackcurrants are, of course, seasonal in their fresh form. These have not been included in this elimination procedure, which has been devised for use at any time of the year. These fruits should be tested when they become available in their normal season.

Complicated manufactured foods, such as jams, confectionary, sauces, cakes, biscuits, gravies, pizzas and alcoholic drinks are mostly mixtures of items already tested, such as sugar, wheat, corn, yeast, soy and egg. If you have this sort of food sensitivity you will have problems with manufactured foods unless you have neutralisation therapy (see chapter 6). These foods may also contain certain chemicals which have been tested, such as anti-staling agents, monosodium glutamate, and aspartame. They can also contain various food dyes, for example, which have not yet been tested. Should you find yourself reacting to a food containing multiple ingredients you know you are usually safe with, it is more than likely that you are reacting to one of the chemical additives.

At the end of Stage 3 you should, therefore, have found what is perhaps best termed a 'compatible diet'. Most people will have found that of the 84 items tested, 79 or more are satisfactory. For people who eat mostly at home, avoidance may be a practical consideration, particularly if they can find less commonly eaten foods to substitute for foods like wheat. All of the major supermarket chains now stock an excellent range of 'free from' foods as do the many health food shops. For those people who have to eat out a lot in the course of their occupation, neutralisation may be desirable (see chapter 6).

There are, of course, many excellent foods not tested on the above 84-food test regime, but anyone who has been through that regime will know how to go about food testing, and any of these items can now be tested and added to your repertoire. I include a list of such foods (see Table 5.3), largely to jog your memory.

Table 5.3 Foods not included in Stages 1–3 of the elimination diet

Vegetables

Brussel sprouts	
Artichokes	Aubergines
Beans, including:	Bamboo shoots
aduki	Celeriac
butter (lima)	Chicory
broad (fava)	Kelp
kidney	Okra
Garden cress	Gherkins
Other peas, including:	Pumpkin
black-eyed	Radishes

chick-peas (garbanzo)
split peas
Squashes (various)
Yams

Sago palm
Salsify

Fowl
Grouse
Guinea fowl
Pheasant
Pigeon
Quail

Meats
Rabbit
Hare

Fruits
Apricots
Blackberries
Blueberries
Cantaloupe
Cherries
Clementines
Crab apples
Cranberries
Elderberries
Gooseberries
Kiwi fruit
Limes
Loganberries
Mandarins
Mangoes
Nectarines
Pomegranates
Prunes
Raspberries
Satsumas
Strawberries

Nuts
Almonds
Brazil nuts
Chestnuts
Filberts
Hazelnuts
Pecans
Walnuts

Grains
Buckwheat
Millet
Wild rice

Tangerines
Ugli fruit

Shellfish
Cockles
Crab
Cray fish
Lobster
Mussels
Oysters
Scallops
Whelks
Winkles

Salt and freshwater fish
Anchovies

Brill	Sardines
Carp	Herring
Caviar	Sole
Eel	Squid / octopus
Halibut	Swordfish
Huss	Turbot
Mullet	Whitebait
Perch	Whiting

Miscellaneous
Herbal tea (different herbs separately, though any reaction is very unlikely)
Green tea
China tea
Goats' milk
Sheeps' milk
Rhubarb
Arrowroot

This list of foods does not contain the enormous range of individual herbs and spices which is available. It also does not contain many occasionally available foods. Various exotic fish and tropical fruits, for example, are now available in markets and restaurants. These foods can gradually be reintroduced into your diet at your leisure. Many people, especially those with very conservative eating habits, will probably eat hardly any of these items prior to a food sensitivity investigation. The general attitude of doctors in this field is, however, to encourage their patients to eat as wide a range of foods as possible. As sensitivity seems to relate to the frequency of eating specific foods, the less frequently any individual food is consumed the more likely you are to remain tolerant to it. To prevent the development of further food sensitivities, therefore, you should make a point of eating a wide range of foods and varying them as much as possible (see chapter 4).

Many people, when they first attended my clinic, told me proudly that they ate very simply and never varied their diet. They considered it a virtue, but they were, in fact wrong; it was probably the main reason why they needed to see me in the first place.

Troubleshooting

Completing the three stages of my elimination diet can take up to six weeks. It can take another two more weeks if you react to several foods, because you have to wait for a reaction to subside. This can often take two days. In the period of six to eight weeks lots of thing can happen in your social or business life:

- You may be invited to an important social event and get carried away with all the food and drink on offer.
- You may need to stay overnight in a hotel, which can frequently mean losing control of what you are eating.
- An unexpected crisis may develop in your life making it difficult or impossible to concentrate on your diet for a week or more.

All of the above, or any other situation, can lead you astray and result in weight gain and possibly the return of any symptoms you might have lost.

When I was in practice these circumstances usually led to 'phone calls of the, 'Help – what should I do now?' variety. Firstly, these situations are not the end of the diet and there is no need to have to start all over again. At the same time, obviously, the later in the diet that this happens the better it is.

If the problem was caused by a social event that lasted only one day, all you need to do is to return to the foods that had been passed as safe up to that point. Usually any weight gain, and symptoms, will disappear in 48 hours. If you have been off the diet for a week or more it usually takes about five days of returning to your 'safe' foods before your weight will return to its previously lower level, and any symptoms will disappear.

'For how long will I need to avoid a food I am sensitive to?'

Many people find that if they avoid a food they have discovered causes a problem for between six months and two years they can eat it once again without any consequences. It's not uncommon for people to find that they can eat most foods after two years, or often much less, but the odd one or possibly two foods may still remain a problem for some time. However, you may decide that in the grand scheme of things a transient rise in weight for a few days is a small price to pay for enjoying a particular food.

The important point to grasp is that you can become tolerant of a food in a comparatively short space of time. However, don't be misled into thinking you were wrong in the first place because if you start eating it again on a regular basis the sensitivity will come galloping back.

Lists of foods containing wheat, corn, milk, yeast and soy can be found in appendix I.

Food content of alcoholic beverages

All alcoholic beverages except spirits contain yeast. Spirits are distilled and most if not all the yeast is lost in this process. Thus whisky, vodka, gin and rum are yeast free.

Wines including champagne all contain yeast, grapes and chemicals such sulphites, and usually anti-staling agents. Cheap wines can contain a lot of these chemicals, which explains why some people react badly to cheap wines but not to the more expensive ones. Red wine contains tannin, not present in white wine.

All beers contain yeast and various grains. Most whisky is made from wheat but bourbon whiskey is made from corn. Vodka is usually made from wheat but some cheaper varieties use potatoes. Gin is made from various grains and spices. Rum is always made from cane sugar.

Fortified wines like sherry, cinzano, port and brandy are a mixture of wine and spirit. Liqueurs are similar. All these drinks are complex.

When/if you find the underlying foods are not incriminated in your weight/health problems, the associated drinks can be tested, bearing in mind the additional ingredients mentioned above. Dry white wine can be tested on day 17 (see page 62) if grapes and yeast are not a problem. You can alternatively try red wine if you prefer, but taking into account the additional presence of tannins. Again, if cane sugar passes the test (day 24) you can try Jamaican rum with soda or a pure fruit juice, such as pineapple (allowed from day 1).

When all the basics have been sorted out you have a choice of either contacting individual manufacturers or just going for 'suck it and see'.

Chapter 6

Desensitisation to food sensitivities

To desensitise or not?

At the end of the elimination diet there comes the decision whether or not it is feasible to avoid the incriminated foods. If you have completed your diet and find that you are sensitive to, for example, coffee and eggs, it is quite easy to avoid these foods. Almost everyone with this relatively simple degree of problem will elect to do so. Even if coffee has been a major part of your existence for some time, it is surprising, particularly when you realise what damage it has been causing, how soon you can come to regard your best friend as your worst enemy. Do not forget, in this particular circumstance the main reason you so needed the coffee resulted from the masking effect (as described on page 41).

The decision to avoid or to desensitise must be right for you. There is, for example, a world of difference between a retired person who doesn't eat out frequently and prepares most of his/her own meals and a person who works in a big city in a job that involves a lot of entertaining clients.

I vividly remember the case of one of my early patients who had severe migraine – about two per week. On the elimination diet he reacted only to corn. I saw him two to three months later about something else and asked him how his migraines were. Ruefully he told me they were as bad as ever. In an average meal in an expensive restaurant, corn may easily be included in most dishes in various forms. However, the stress of the question and answer session with the waiter in front of potential or important clients made it impractical to identify which dishes might be risky. Soon he had given up the struggle and gone back to having migraines. I told him about desensitisation and after 30 minutes of skin testing we were able to make up his 'vaccine'. By taking this he was then able to eat normally and still be migraine free. Three years later he told me that the 30 minutes we had spent skin testing him had revolutionised his whole life.

You need to read the rest of this detailed chapter only if you are interested in being desensitised. From the outset you must be aware that it will involve giving yourself tiny, under-the-skin injections every other day (or drops under the tongue three times a day) with the appropriate vaccine for two years or more.

Most patients are a little apprehensive about injecting themselves. The needles used in desensitisation are in fact both short and very fine, as used by diabetics for insulin. The injections are normally put into the large thigh muscles. To demonstrate how minimal the procedure is I pinch the patient's leg, tell them to look away, and then ask if I have given the injection. Normally they say 'no', at which point I tell them to look back and to their surprise the needle is in their leg and they haven't felt a thing. I then ask them to give themselves the injection while they are still sat with me.

I have found about 2 % of patients to be mega needle phobic and in these people I offer desensitisation treatment sublingually (under the tongue). They need to place one drop of the desensitising solution from a pipette under their tongue three times daily. This certainly works in some, but not all, patients. In practice, this form of the treatment can be a real pain in the neck as the drops only work for about five hours as opposed to 48 hours by injection. To ensure that only one drop is administered it is also necessary always to carry a mirror as well as the drops.

Some people think that if a food is 'bad' for them then it is surely better for them to avoid it even if it is difficult to do so.

When I first encountered this subject I felt very much the same. However, as time passed I changed my mind. Most people do very well with desensitisation and are able to lead an entirely normal life, eating-wise. Eliminating such items as coffee or sugar has no detrimental effect on general health, but avoiding a wide range of foods such as cereal grains and dairy is not to be recommended as it can lead to nutritional deficiencies.

The other problem is that someone who is sensitive to wheat, corn, oats, rye and malt will usually start eating lots of potatoes, sweet potatoes and rice as an alternative. This may work well for a long time, but may in some people lead to them becoming sensitive to one of these alternative foods. For example, if a person has been eating potatoes four times a week without problems for many years, eating them six times a week may lead to him/her becoming sensitised to them.

The discovery of desensitisation

Allergists who have worked for years giving patients arbitrary and increasing doses of injected allergens for inhaled allergy problems have known that occasionally patients would report a startling improvement in their condition within an hour or so of receiving an allergy injection. This improvement would often last several days. Such patients would often return and ask for a further injection (exactly the same as the last one). This rapid relief puzzled most such allergists, who considered it to be a psychological quirk.

However, in 1957 Dr Carleton H. Lee of Kansas, Missouri, made the discovery which explained this curious phenomenon, and opened up the most amazing vista for the control of sensitivity responses to foods, inhaled allergens, chemicals and even hormones and viruses. Dr Lee's wife had severe asthma which he had discovered was related to the consumption of certain foods. Unfortunately, she reacted to a huge range and could remain well only on two or three specific foods. Other foods would quickly bring on moderate or severe asthmatic attacks within a few hours.

Although food extract injection therapy had never before been found to have any use, Dr Lee persisted in experimenting with injecting food extracts in the hope of helping his wife's problem. He eventually discovered to his delight that he could produce asthmatic symptoms with one carefully measured dose of food extract injected intradermally (between the layers of the skin). More importantly, he found that another specific concentration would relieve this asthma within 10 minutes. This specific dose that relieved symptoms became known as the 'desensitising dose'. He then went on to observe that this specific dose, when given by a small subcutaneous injection (just under the skin), would protect his wife for the next two or three days should she eat that particular food. A cocktail of all the desensitising doses of the foods to which she was sensitive, administered in a single injection about three times a week, would enable her to eat normally without any asthma.

Thus was born 'provocational desensitising' testing and treatment. The word 'provocation' refers to the production of symptoms with one dose of the injected allergen. The term 'desensitisation' relates to the relief of symptoms with a weaker dose. Desensitisation therapy is the treatment of the problem by low, tailor-made doses of the foods to which you are sensitive. This is most effectively administered by subcutaneous injection. Administration can also be done with sublingual (under the tongue) drops, but, as already explained, is usually more effective if given by injection.

Soon Dr Lee discovered that he could utilise the same principles to 'neutralise' reactions to inhaled allergens such as house dust, dust mites, moulds, animal furs and summer pollens. It had been possible to treat such problems before with conventional incremental desensitisation, but the success rate was low (often below

20%) and the treatment took months or years to work. (While neutralisation (desensitisation) for inhaled allergies is very effective I have never found weight problems to be caused by inhalants.)

Safety of this form of desensitisation

In 1986 in the UK, desensitisation treatment suddenly made the headlines in the national press. The Committee on Safety in Medicines, a government-appointed watchdog on the pharmaceutical industry, ruled that **conventional incremental desensitisation** should be administered only by doctors working in units where there was adequate resuscitative equipment and the knowledge to use it. Furthermore, they ruled that patients were to remain in the units for an hour or so after testing until it was quite certain that no adverse response to the injection would occur.

Up to the time of this ruling, most of the incremental desensitising injections had been given rather casually in doctors' surgeries, and often the patient had been allowed to go home immediately. Many GPs had not been well trained in how to deal with the adverse reactions that these injections had often initiated. As a result of this situation there had been, over the previous few years, a handful of patients who had died as a result of this type of treatment. All of these patients were severe asthmatics who are amongst the most difficult patients to treat in the whole field of allergic practice.

As a result of the 1986 ruling, incremental desensitisation virtually stopped in the UK, except in a few allergy units in National Health Service hospitals. Although the safety of incremental desensitisation was probably higher than that of many drugs, such as anti-inflammatory drugs used by the million for treating arthritis, the benefit/risk ratio was low. That is, fewer than 20% of patients benefit from incremental desensitisation to allergens such as house dust, dust mites and moulds. The success rate with incremental desensitisation to animal furs is even lower. Summer pollen incremental desensitisation is more successful, but the season is limited. Summer problems are usually less of a strain on patients than allergens which affect them all year round, such as house dust.

In contrast, **provocative desensitisation (neutralisation) therapy has proved to be totally safe.** There has not, to my knowledge, been a single fatality recorded anywhere in the world as a result of this type of testing or therapy. All doctors practising provocative desensitisation, however, do carry full resuscitative equipment as a precaution. Currently there are about six clinics using this method in the UK, compared with several hundred in the USA. Provocative desensitisation is used as a method of choice by members of the American Academy of Environmental Medicine, the American Academy of Otolaryngolic Allergy and the Pan American Allergy Society. The combined membership of these large societies exceeds 5,000 and all run annual instructional courses for physicians interested in the technique. In the UK these courses are run by the British Society for Ecological Medicine. Many ENT specialists in the USA use desensitisation as the treatment of choice for rhinitis and related conditions.

In the UK, my clinic pioneered provocative desensitisation testing in 1977, but many American clinics had been using it prior to that. Dr Lee made his initial observations in 1957 and treated many patients in the years after. Professor Joseph Miller became interested in 1965 and had gained so much experience in it by 1972 that he was ready to publish his book *Food Allergy: Provocative Testing and Injection Therapy*. This became the 'bible' for many American allergists who started treating patients in this manner soon after. In 1987 Lee published a further definitive book about his technique, entitled *Allergy Neutralization: The Lee Method*. Later, Professor Miller wrote the book entitled *Relief at Last: Neutralization for Food Allergy and Other Illnesses*. There have been many clinical trials validating this method.[8–18]

At a conservative estimate, at least 25 million patients have received this form of treatment over a period of many years, without any fatalities. Most of these patients were in the USA or Canada, but several hundred thousand were treated in the UK or Australia.

This safety record is not surprising when one considers that the provocative desensitisation method uses doses that are frequently several thousand times weaker than those used in incremental desensitisation. Furthermore, the tailor-made doses employed for provocative desensitisation are ones which:

- have a completely negative skin reaction;
- have an immediate positive health benefit.

In 1987 the Committee on Safety in Medicines acknowledged that their strictures concerning incremental desensitisation did not apply to low-dose desensitisation therapy. They had not considered provocative desensitisation in their deliberations as there had been no problems reported.

The technique

Food extracts are obtained from the usual supply companies in the standard 1/10 or 1/20 prick test concentrations containing glycerine. These are usually administered by a specialist nurse. The glycerine is added during the initial extraction process to stabilise the food extract so that it maintains its potency for many years. The dilutant that most clinics use nowadays is benzyl alcohol, as it has a very low incidence of allergy itself. The benzyl alcohol is prepared in intravenous-quality normal saline. Using this dilutant, nine separate dilutions are prepared; each one being a fifth of the strength of the previous one. Thus dilutions of 1/5, 1/25, 1/125, 1/625 and so on are prepared for testing.

The test consists of giving intradermal injections of varying concentrations of the food known or suspected to be causing the patient's problems. Testing usually begins with the 1/5 strength, and if a positive reaction on the skin is obtained we then proceed at 10-minute intervals to progressively weaker strengths.

When 0.05 cm^3 of a food extract is injected intradermally it will produce a wheal, which at the time of injection is hard, raised and blanched (white) and has well-demarcated edges. It usually measures 7 mm in diameter. In assessing wheals there are various criteria. After 10 minutes a positive wheal will usually have retained most of these features and have grown at least 2 mm in diameter. Negative wheals lose these characteristics and grow less than 2 mm.

If the initial injection results in a positive wheal, with or without symptoms, the nurse moves to a consecutively weaker strength until the first negative wheal is found. This is the de-sensitisation dose and also the correct concentration to be used for treatment, unless symptoms induced by the greater strength have not entirely cleared, in which case a move to the next weaker solution will normally clear them. In over 90% of cases the first negative wheal signals the desensitising dose. If a weaker dose than the desensitising one is administered, then symptoms will usually recur. This is called under-dosage and the symptoms will be removed by going back to the stronger dose, which is obviously the desensitising level. Thus, in someone suffering from headaches, for example, a headache can be induced by too strong or too weak a dose, but can be removed by the desensitis-ing dose. Many people find it amazing that all their symptoms can be turned on and off within a few minutes. They often find the changes so impressive that they wish medical sceptics could observe the changes they are experiencing in their bodies. People who are just overweight with no symptoms develop no symp-toms on testing, but still get the skin reactions

In 1985 there was a BBC TV *Horizon* broadcast on the topic of food allergy, watched by over 11 million people. The pro-gramme opened with a video recording of an American physi-cian with severe arthritis, who had been treated by Dr Marshall Mandell, who practises in New England. It showed a short sequence of this severely arthritic doctor walking with obvious pain and difficulty. Several minutes later, after a desensitising injection had been given, this very same doctor was able to walk easily and with virtually no pain. Later in the same programme I showed a female patient with rheumatoid arthritis having pain induced in her hands with a 1/25 extract of wheat, followed by total relief a few minutes later after an injection of 1/625 extract of wheat. The programme evoked a great deal of interest on the part of the general public, but sadly very little from the medical profession, who appear to lack curiosity about these interesting phenomena.

These techniques do, after all, lend themselves to fairly simple scientific evaluation. The patient has no way of knowing whether a testing nurse or physician is using an active ingredient or a dummy 'placebo' injection of, for example, normal saline. I have frequently demonstrated to physicians visiting my clinic that patients can identify from their clinical responses whether they are being injected with one of their known allergens or a placebo. These same physicians are usually highly impressed and often go off to do the same work themselves. However, until the higher echelons of the medical profession, the teaching hospital professors and so forth, become interested, dissemination of this knowledge is going to be painfully slow. In the meantime, millions of patients with a wide variety of symptoms/conditions caused by food sensitivity are going to continue to suffer.

To anyone reading this who thinks it might just be a placebo effect, I would like to point out that provocative desensitisation is just as effective on animals. In 1992 I participated in a clinical study to test desensitisation on horses[7] with a leading vet in the Epsom area. He now uses this technique for horses with asthma, urticaria and head shaking. In a study he conducted,[7] over 80% of horses with these conditions improved dramatically. As far as I am aware horses don't hold any preconceived ideas as to the value or otherwise of their treatment! Clinical trials have, however, been performed on desensitisation therapy in humans and these have been published in various journals. There have, in fact been around 15 trials of desensitisation testing and therapy published. All but one have been positive in their conclusions. The one exception was organised by an orthopaedic surgeon rather than an allergist. In this study there were countless mistakes.

Food avoidance

It is important to be sure the therapy is working for all the foods for which it has been sought. Therefore, when you start your injections (one daily for the first two weeks) you should avoid the 'guilty' foods for the first three days. After that, each food should be re-introduced, one per day. Once the food has been found no longer to cause problems, it can be eaten regularly thereafter. Occasionally you may find that desensitisation works for a number of foods but not for one in particular.

How desensitiation therapy works

Currently we know a certain amount about the immunological process that is involved in the desensitisation phenomenon. The fine details, however, are not fully understood and I think it may well be many years before they are. The same problem applies to many medical treatments currently available:

- we do not know how painkillers work
- we do not know how sleeping tablets work
- we do not know how some tranquilisers work
- we do not know how anti-inflammatory drugs work in relieving the pain and swelling in arthritis
- we do not know how gold injections work in rheumatoid arthritis
- we do not know how conventional incremental desensitisation works (or does not work!)

I could go on for long time in this vein. Most drug treatment has been discovered by chance in an empirical fashion. New drugs are usually found by trying out a whole range of new synthetic chemicals on animals such as guinea pigs and rats. Those which appear to have the more beneficial effect are tried out on 'higher' animals, such as cats. After animal experimentation, the more promising-looking drugs are then tried on human volunteers. The whole process is therefore based much more on trial and error than on any great understanding of the underlying mechanism of the disease process that is being considered.

In order to give some idea as to how desensitisation works, it is necessary to enter the world of immunology. This is complicated and you may wish to skip the science and move on to 'Administration of desensitisation' on page 89.

In an immune response we have on the one hand allergenic molecules (the particles that make up the substance producing the allergic reaction), and on the other, the organs in the body which react to them. The organ that produces the reaction is called a stress organ. In the case of, for example, arthritis, the stress organ is the joint or joints, or perhaps more precisely, the lining of the joints.

Allergenic molecules of food or inhalants cause reactions in stress organs through two types of cell - 'mast cells' and 'basophils'. These cells release histamine granules and other potentially harmful chemicals. Mast cells were called such because under the microscope they look like bags of mast (nuts, seeds and acorns). Mast cells are found on the outer surface of the capillaries (the smallest blood vessels) just under the skin, or around the capillaries in the lining of the respiratory or digestive tracts. Mast cells cling to the capillaries like a great swarm of bees clinging to the branches of a tree.

Basophils, in contrast, normally reside in the bloodstream itself and circulate around the whole body. When necessary, basophils have the ability to enter tissues through breaks in the capillary blood vessels. They can then release their granules and other chemicals to help the effects of their sister cells, the mast cells. The chemicals, particularly histamine, released by these two types of cells cause the allergic reaction. Other chemicals they release, called 'prostaglandins' and 'leucotrienes', can be quite harmful as they can, in turn, stimulate other types of cell to arrive at the reaction site. These other cells release further potentially harmful chemicals to fight the original cause of the problem. These other chemicals are more difficult to overcome. This mechanism increases the response to the problem substance, but these extra chemicals may well cause the destruction of normal tissue. Thus the reaction changes from a purely allergic response to an inflammation.

The chemical mediators released from mast cells and basophils can occur not only as a reaction to allergic molecules, but also as a reaction to viral infections, excessive cold, and certain hormonal changes.

The skin is composed of two layers, the epidermis (outer layer) and dermis (inner layer). When an intradermal ('between the layers') injection is administered, it stimulates the vast network of highly reactive immunological cells situated in the skin. Allergens injected into the epidermis can make the mast cells surrounding the capillaries sting the capillaries like a bee. The venom from this 'sting' (chemical mediators) forces the local capillaries, which are only one cell thick, to contract and become slightly separated from each other, opening up tiny crevices between them.

The gaps so caused allow a two-way flow from the tissues into the capillaries and from the capillaries into the bloodstream. Injected antigen and some chemical mediators enter the bloodstream, and watery blood serum containing basophils and chemical leaks into the tissues while the reaction is occurring.

This increased flow between the capillaries and the surrounding tissue is critical to allergic or inflammatory reactions. The body can excrete harmful allergens quickly into the bloodstream and deposit them in the tissues where they will be less of a problem. It can send protective substances, such as antibodies, quickly out of the bloodstream through these capillary gaps.

Desensitisation occurs when homeostatic balance is achieved in this two-way process. Immunologists are learning that these homeostatic controlling mechanisms are incredibly complex and numerous. There are many factors stimulating or suppressing reactions.

The immune system is like a million huge armies that have many weapons and strategies co-ordinated to oppose similarly huge armies of allergens, bacteria, viruses, fungi, yeasts and toxins.

The dose of the offending substance that is given in desensitisation therapy drives the system back towards a normal balance – 'homeostasis'. This usually occurs within a few minutes, turning off the release of the harmful histamines and the other chemical mediators much more quickly and effectively than any other known technique.

Administration of desensitisation

After the desensitising levels of the major food sensitivities have been determined, desensitisation therapy can be self-administered either by sublingual drops or by intradermal (under the skin) injections. As explained earlier, sublingual drops are so called because they are placed beneath the tongue. The skin under the human tongue is an area of high absorbability, and inspection will reveal large veins (the 'sublingual veins'). This is why patients who are taking nitroglycerine tablets to treat angina place these tablets under their tongue to obtain the most rapid response. Technicians use a fairly simple mathematical formula to calculate the level each patient needs, depending on the results of skin-testing.

Diagnosis using skin-testing

An extension of provocative desensitisation is to use it for diagnosis. Clearly, if positive wheal reactions and symptoms can be obtained in the course of desensitisation, there is no need to go through the process of an elimination diet. Furthermore, whereas a full elimination dietary procedure can take five or six weeks, during which time you have to avoid major social occasions, a comprehensive skin-testing programme can be completed in about three days of intensive testing (six sessions of 2½ hours). A workable procedure here is to scan about 34 foods in intradermal provocational tests. The reaction to all 34 foods is assessed, and desensitising doses obtained for all of the items to which there is a positive reaction. At the end of the testing programme, you are allowed to eat only those foods tested and take injections or drops to cover all of those items to which sensitivity has been found.

The advantages of this approach are considerable, including:
- The testing programme is completed in a few days
- You do not have to assess your own response
- You do not have to abandon any drugs you are taking, which can be either hazardous or extremely unpleasant for some people
- If you live a long way from the clinic, this test procedure saves a whole series of long journeys
- If you have multiple food sensitivities, these tests will be inevitable anyway, even after the elimination diet, because you may need to be desensitised to a large number of foods
- In most cases the treatment is very successful.

The disadvantages of this treatment, as opposed to the elimination diet followed by desensitisation to specifically identified food sensitivities, are:

- The skin-test technique picks up adapted food sensitivities as well as non-adapted sensitivities (see chapter 4). Hence the number of foods to which someone reacts often appears more complicated than it really is, and a degree of over-treatment is almost inevitable using this technique.
- You do not know that you are going to experience significant weight loss until after the treatment has been completed, whereas after the first stage of the elimination diet most people can discover for themselves that, once the foods that cause the biggest problem are removed from their diet they start steadily losing weight.
- Going through an elimination diet probably gives you a better idea than skin-testing as to which foods cause significant weight gain and those which cause only a minor weight response.
- The elimination diet is an educative programme, whereas skin-testing is far less so in itself. Consequently, at the end of a skin-testing programme you must initially restrict your diet to those foods that have been tested and found 'innocent' and to those foods for which, although positive, you are taking desensitisation.

After remaining on the foods tested for a few weeks and presumably losing weight, you can extend your list of foods eaten by bringing back into your diet one single food item at a time to test it.

Disadvantages of desensitisation therapy

One problem that can occur with desensitisation therapy is that after several weeks or months of this treatment the desensitising levels can change. Often the specific reason for this change is inexplicable, but in many cases it appears to be a feature of the progressive desensitisation that is occurring as treatment continues to be administered. What normally happens is that someone who has experienced dramatic or considerable weight loss suddenly notices the weight is beginning to creep back again without any obvious change in their diet. In these circumstances retesting is necessary. Another possible reason for a change in the desensitisation levels is the occurrence of a severe attack of flu or other similar viral illness. Most frequently the retesting reveals that the desensitising levels have become stronger. In other words, as individuals become progressively desensitised, they need a stronger dose to prevent the weight reaction. It is, furthermore, possible that several months later the desensitisation levels will again change to an even stronger level, at which point the levels usually remain very stable. Certainly, instability of desensitising levels almost inevitably decreases with time.

The main disadvantage with changing desensitising levels concerns the inevitable cost to the patient of retesting and, where necessary, taking time off work for this to be done. If only a few foods are involved this is a minor problem.

The other problem occasionally occurring with desensitisation therapy is that we see some people who cannot be desensitised to one specific food. They may find that the technique works for perhaps four foods, but does not work for the fifth. If any food is going to be a problem it is usually wheat, and this is thought to be because wheat is particularly complex. If, however, the patient can be desensitised to rye (which is usually the case) it provides a reasonably good alternative.

Practical considerations

You may need to think about the following:

- At the end of an elimination diet you need to decide whether simply to avoid problem foods or to use desensitisation.

- If you are sensitive to, say, just coffee and eggs, both are reasonably easy to avoid; however, you will need to become familiar with all the foods that contain them.
- Desensitisation involves a self-administered micro-injection just under the skin, once every other day.
- To determine your specific desensitising levels for each problem food, you will need to attend a clinic providing this service (see appendix II). The clinic will test you with various concentrations of the relevant food to determine your personal desensitising levels.
- On average, it takes about two and a half hours (one session) to obtain desensitising levels for five foods.
- Your personal vaccine will then be made in the laboratory of your clinic.
- When you first receive your personal vaccine my advice is to have an injection daily for the first two weeks. For the first three days, the 'guilty' foods should be avoided, after which each food should be reintroduced, one per day. Once the food has been found no longer to cause problems it can be eaten thereafter. Occasionally you may find a number of foods being tolerated very satisfactorily but one not.
- If you would like to use desensitisation but really cannot handle micro-injections you can try sublingual drops taken three times daily. It is very important to take these correctly and even then they are usually less effective than micro-injections.
- Both the skin testing and the desensitising injections are totally safe. There have been no reported fatalities anywhere. The Burghwood Clinic (Banstead, Surrey) has been using this technique since I opened it in 1982, but I originally started using the technique in 1978. The only patients that need close monitoring are severe asthmatics.
- For some people after a few months of successful

desensitisation things may appear to go wrong. This will be because their personal desensitisation levels have changed for one or more food, at which point their weight may start increasing, and any other symptoms previously eliminated may return. A quick return to the clinic for retesting of levels and a new vaccine usually solves the problem in a few days.

- The cost of the vaccine is usually quite cheap (approx £5 per food item in 2012 in the UK) and lasts for three months. Thus, in the UK desensitisation for five food items for a year would cost around £100, plus a few pounds for the syringes.
- The cost of the skin testing sessions will vary from clinic to clinic. You are advised to ring the clinic in advance to ascertain the current cost. If you know precisely which foods you need desensitising to, obviously this will be cheaper.
- Most people only need to take the vaccine for approximately three years before they are completely desensitised.

Chapter 7

The yeast syndrome and weight problems

The yeast syndrome

Most people who go on a diet excluding all the common food sensitivities notice a huge difference in their weight after seven or eight days. They may also feel greatly improved in their health, often after suffering a distinct withdrawal reaction during the evening of the first day of the diet that continues over the next three to five days before improving. A minority may observe no weight loss other than perhaps a couple of pounds (1 kg) due to the restricted diet. They may also have no withdrawal symptoms and find no improvement in their health after seven days.

What is happening in these disappointing cases? These people may be reacting to yeast or fungal organisms in their gut which can upset their weight-regulating mechanisms, in the same way that individual food sensitivities can. Other possibilities are that they are suffering from low thyroid production (see chapter 8) or problems associated with refined carbohydrates (chapter 10).

Being overweight can thus have multiple causes, and some people may have both food sensitivities *and* the yeast syndrome. Generally you should sort out any food sensitivities first, and then treat the yeast problem.

My first clue to the connection between the yeast syndrome and weight problems came in a series of lectures given by Dr Orion Truss at the 15th Advanced Seminar of the American

Academy of Environmental Medicine, at Pine Mountain near Atlanta, Georgia, USA. The lectures concerned the relationship between the yeast, *Candida albicans* (otherwise known as 'thrush'), and human illness.

Thrush is a condition that most people have heard about. Up to the time of this meeting, I had thought of *Candida albicans* as causing only vaginal thrush in women and oral thrush, most frequently in the mouths of babies. Both conditions are usually cured by short courses of fungicides and – except in a few unfortunate women where the condition may recur with monotonous regularity – were not thought of as a major problem.

What Dr Orion Truss said was that this view was wrong and that *intestinal* thrush could cause a huge array of medical problems, varying quite considerably in symptom pattern from one person to another. He also said that the problem was extremely common and was a major cause of human illness.

Dr Truss is, I might add, a physician of considerable standing and has served as Instructor in Medicine at Cornell Medical College and Instructor in Clinical Medicine at the University of Alabama Medical College, amongst other major appointments.

What this physician had in fact discovered was another basic cause of illness. Not only could people respond adversely to the foods, chemicals and inhalants that they encountered, but they could also react to the microflora of their intestinal tract.

Having spent many years researching the role of candidiasis in human illness, Dr Truss reported his observations in three separate papers in the *Journal of Orthomolecular Medicine*. These papers did not make a great impact on the medical profession in general, mostly I think because physicians could not perceive how these findings could fit in with their other knowledge and medical practice. However, physicians in the allergy field who were looking at illness purely in terms of cause and effect, as opposed to naming a disease and attempting to suppress it, knew they had been missing a major cause of illness, and so this work fell on much more receptive ears in their case.

At this point I must emphasise that in my experience direct problems with internal candidiasis play a major part in understanding weight problems.

The yeast phenomenon

Like most of life, the whole yeast problem centres around balance. On one side of the equation are one or more types of yeast, and on the other side is the resistance of the host, that is, *you*.

Although *Candida* has in the past been regarded as an innocent inhabitant of the digestive tract, mycology (the study of moulds and fungi) has demonstrated that *Candida albicans* is very complex. It releases at least 79 known chemical substances, against which the human body creates an identifiable antibody. To complicate matters, there are in fact 81 strains of *Candida albicans*, and each strain can produce 35 separate antigens. Varying strains can colonise the gut of the same person at different times in his or her life. Healthy individuals have these organisms present only in small quantities in their gastrointestinal tract, and in such people no harm results.

Yeasts and fungi are opportunistic organisms. They will grow spectacularly when an individual's resistance is lowered or when they are particularly encouraged by certain factors. Resistance can be lowered by an infection, nutritional deficiencies, or some debilitating agent in the environment. Factors in our modern lifestyle that are important are high consumption of antibiotics, the contraceptive pill, and cortisone. High sugar and yeast consumption are also very important, especially sugar.

Candida albicans can exist in two separate forms and is therefore called a 'dimorphic' organism. When conditions are ripe for its proliferation, it tends to change in shape from its normal yeast-like form to a fungal form. The yeast-like form is thought to be non-invasive and probably harmless. The fungal form, however, has long root-like 'mycelia', which can penetrate the mucous membrane lining of the intestines. This penetration can lead to 'leaky' mucous membranes. Fig. 7.1 shows a drawing of the organism based on a light microscope photograph, with the different elements indicated.

Such a leaky intestinal lining is of enormous importance as it can allow incompletely digested dietary proteins and other foods to come into direct contact with the immune system. The outposts of the immune system lie underneath the intestinal lining and they are designed to deal with food that has been broken down by digestive enzymes and is thus of low molecular weight.

Figure 7.1: Drawing of *Candida albicans* as it appears under a high-resolution light microscope.

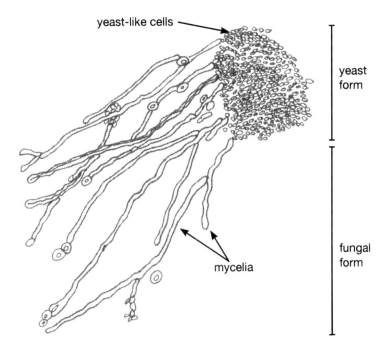

The contact between the immune system and these unbroken-down foodstuffs is an obvious mechanism for the production of food sensitivity. Hence, people who have a chronic over-growth of *Candida albicans,* with a high percentage in the mycelial form, frequently show a wide variety of food and environmental allergies and sensitivities.

People with multiple food sensitivities may be that way because antibodies have formed to the antigenic proteins in foods. In addition to causing a leaky gut lining it has now been convincingly demonstrated that *Candida* produces a specific toxin, not surprisingly called 'Candida toxin', which seems to weaken the immune system in general and make it less able to cope with other allergy problems. In particular, Candida toxin suppresses the T-lymphocytes in our immune defence systems, and as these cells are the 'generals' of the system, the immune system tends to perform in a rather disorganised manner.

It is thought that when neutralisation therapy for food and inhalant allergies and sensitivities is not working as expected (see chapter 6), it is usually because of a poorly functioning immune system and is accompanied by depressed levels of T-lymphocytes. Many failures of neutralisation become successes after *Candida* treatment.

Candida treatment is thought to lead to a reduction in gut permeability, and it is very noticeable clinically that further food sensitivities seem much less likely to occur. In people with multiple, complex health problems and food sensitivities, *Candida* treatment tends to stabilise them and make them easier to treat. Minor food sensitivities often disappear and neutralisation levels remain much more stable.

What is the real cause of the yeast syndrome?

At one time Professor Jonathan Brostoff – who was Head of the Department of Allergy at the Middlesex Hospital in London –

called this problem: 'That syndrome which responds to anti-fungal drugs and a sugar-free, yeast-free diet.'

Dr Keith Eaton, a close friend of mine, spent a great deal of time researching this area and publishing many papers in the *Journal of Nutritional and Environmental Medicine*. Tragically, he died in 2006 without really nailing the culprit.

One possibility is that there are several yeasts other than the various *Candida* species. They include *Torulopsis glabrata*, and *Cryptococcus histolytica*. Any or all of these organisms could be partly responsible as they would respond to the same treatment as *Candida*. Other possibilities include parasites such as *Giardia lamblia* and *Blastocystis hominis*.

I am fairly certain that these parasites are not the cause of this syndrome as they do not respond at all to nystatin, ampho-tericin-B and other anti-yeast medications. The main sticking point with this dilemma is that various yeasts are not reliably present in stool samples. They are certainly present quite often, but not always. This may be due to the fungal or mycelial form of *Candida* described earlier being embedded in the mucous membranes lining the small and large bowels, and not making it down the gut into the stools.

Personally, I tend to think that Dr Orion Truss was right all along, partly because I have seen some very interesting results when intradermal skin testing with extracts of *Candida albicans* manufactured by one of the allergy supply companies. (Intrader-mal testing and desensitisation are described in detail in chapter 6.) Testing with relatively strong doses of *Candida albicans* can induce the person's symptoms, which are then relieved spectac-ularly by giving a weaker neutralising dose.

The gut fermentation test

The best test for this syndrome is called a 'gut fermentation test'. If positive, this test is the best evidence that excess fermentation is occurring in the gut. Excessive fermentation is caused by yeasts.

If a person should have a positive gut fermentation test and/or display various symptoms which I will describe, the probability is further increased. A positive gut fermentation test by itself is pretty good evidence, and ultimately the best way forward is a clinical trial of the appropriate treatment.

At the time of writing, the gut fermentation test is performed in the UK only at the Biolab Medical Unit (see appendix II). They will take referrals from doctors and qualified nutritionists.

For this test, you have to attend in person and abstain from all alcohol for at least 24 hours beforehand. You also have to abstain from all food and drink (except mineral water) for at least three hours before the test.

When you arrive at the laboratory you swallow 2 grams of dextrose in enteric coated capsules washed down with 50 grams of dextrose in 100 ml of water (the 'glucose challenge'). Blood is then drawn for analysis 60 minutes later. In the early days of this test a pre-challenge blood test was always taken, but this was abandoned after all these tests were found to be negative. (The technique employs 'gas liquid chromatography'. The precise details are very complicated and I will not describe them here.)

In people with the 'yeast syndrome', the chief abnormality found is excess ethanol (alcohol) in the blood. Quantities in excess of 22 millimoles (mmol) per litre are regarded as positive and an excellent confirmation of the diagnosis of yeast/fungal syndrome. Sometimes very high levels of ethanol are discovered with this test, which disappear after appropriate treatment.

I must add that a few people who have a strong history of the yeast syndrome will respond to treatment for this despite a negative gut fermentation test.

Finally, I would like to emphasise that whichever yeast is involved in this problem, that yeast stays within the interior or lining of the gut. The symptoms that occur exterior to the gut must be, in my view, some type of sensitivity reaction or a distant effect of the toxins produced by the yeast.

Symptoms particularly suggestive of the yeast syndrome

- Recurring vaginal or penile thrush
- chronic rectal irritation
- recurring bouts of cystitis or urethritis (with no bacteria found in mid-stream specimens of urine)
- recurring depression, irritability, inability to concentrate and problems with memory
- chronic nervous indigestion symptoms in the upper part of the digestive tract, especially with excessive wind and bloating
- chronic constipation, sometimes alternating with diarrhoea
- recurring fungal-type rashes, such as fungal-type eczema, urticaria and psoriasis.

Of importance is the observation that these symptoms may be worse after :
- courses of antibiotics
- courses of the contraceptive pill
- high consumption of sugary products
- high consumption of yeast products such as wine, beer, Marmite, vinegar, leavened (yeast-containing) bread.

When making a diagnosis of the 'yeast syndrome' by symptoms, the doctor is looking for those I have just described, plus a list of predisposing factors in the person's history. This list readily tells us why we are in such a medical mess at the beginning of the 21st century. It also gives most of the clues as to why obesity has been increasing at something like 8% over each decade for the last 40 years.

The 'yeast syndrome' is thought by many physicians to pre-dispose to food sensitivity; certainly many people I have seen who have multiple food sensitivities stop developing new sensitivities after treatment for the yeast syndrome.

Factors predisposing to the yeast syndrome

Recurrent or prolonged treatment with antibiotics

Antibiotics were first discovered in 1939, but not used extensively until the mid-1940s. Later they were used, not only on doctors' prescription, but also in rearing animals. All physicians know (or should know) that antibiotics stir up intestinal thrush and similar yeasts. What they usually don't appreciate are the long-term effects that can accrue.

The worst in this respect are the broad spectrum antibiotics such as tetracycline. These antibiotics kill a lot of the more innocent micro-organisms in the digestive tract, and thereby encourage yeasts and fungi to flourish as the competing powerful bacteria are partially eradicated.

The worst single example of this is the current prevalent practice of treating teenage acne with prolonged courses of tetracycline, often extending over several years. I have seen many healthy teenagers (apart from the acne) converted to medical wrecks after two years of consuming broad spectrum antibiotics. Symptoms such as depression, fatigue, headaches, migraine and obesity can result. The antibiotics are usually prescribed by dermatologists, but the fallout is dealt with by psychiatrists, and neurologists and non-dermatologists – one of the great dangers of medical specialisation where the left hand doesn't know what the right hand is doing.

Prolonged use of the contraceptive pill

The contraceptive pill for women was discovered in the mid-1950s and has been used extensively since the early 1960s. Many women develop vaginal thrush soon after starting to take it. Quite how the 'Pill' produces this effect is not well understood, but there is little doubt that it does. Many women also notice large gains in weight. However, in some women, the weight gain is more subtle, starting after several months.

Having stirred up the yeasts, the overgrowth, and related symptoms, may not go into reverse when the woman stops taking the Pill. This is not scientifically proven, but could well be what is happening.

High sugar consumption

In both the UK and the USA, at the beginning of the 20th century, the consumption of sugar was approximately 80 lb (36 kg) of sugar per person per year. Now it is around 144 lb (65.5 kg) per person per year in the UK and 168 lb (76 kg) per person in the USA. In 1850 it was virtually nil in either of these countries except for the very rich. Consumption of other refined carbohydrates like white flour and white bread has also increased. This is by far the largest dietary change that has occurred in the western world in the last two centuries.

Ingestion of yeast products

Yeasts started to be used by human beings 8000 years ago, but only in a small way. Scrumpy (apple cider) was, I understand, one of the earliest examples in Britain. Nowadays yeast products occur prolifically in our diets – yeast is present in all leavened breads, all wines, beer, most cheeses, mushrooms and many fruit juices.

All alcoholic beverages start off as fermented items such as wine. However, spirits such as gin, vodka, whisky and rum are then distilled and almost all the yeast is lost during the distillation process. Hence most spirits are yeast free and people sensitive to yeasts can tolerate them with no or minimal problems. However, if the person is sensitive to wheat s/he will react to Scotch whisky and most vodkas as they are made from wheat.

Other predisposing factors for the yeast syndrome

Other predisposing factors did exist before 1900, and include:
- multiple pregnancies
- moulds: an environment containing a high proportion of moulds.

Moulds
There is a fascinating interaction between environmental moulds and the yeast syndrome. People with severe yeast problems are frequently noticeably worse in the mould season of the year.

Moulds can be divided into indoor moulds and outdoor moulds.

Indoor moulds usually occur in damp conditions and are often visible in bathrooms and kitchens. They can be reduced substantially by the use of retardant sprays which are available in most hardware stores. Another source of indoor moulds is damp soil if you have a large number of pot plants.

Outdoor moulds are pretty well impossible to avoid short of emigrating to hot dry climates, especially desert climates like Arizona and Southern California. In the UK the times of the year when the problem is at its worst is during hot humid days in August, September and early October. During these times the mould count is very high and can be measured. The only thing that can directly help people with mould sensitivity is desensitisation to individual moulds, as is described in chapter 6. Aggressive treatment for the yeast syndrome may also help in the long run.

Treatment of the yeast syndrome

This treatment can often be easy, with spectacular benefits occurring in the first two or three weeks, and people saying they haven't felt so well for 20 years. Other people may find it a slow grind before they improve. Doctors usually use one of the following methods:

- Nystatin plus diet
- Amphoterecin-B plus diet
- Fluconazole (Diflucan) or itraconazole (Sporanox) plus diet.

Other health practitioners use:
- Caprylic acid plus diet
- *Lactobacillus acidophilus* plus diet.

The yeast syndrome can be quite resistant to treatment; the object of the diet is, of course, to deprive the yeast of what it likes to consume. The absolutely ideal diet to combat the yeast syndrome would contain no carbohydrates at all. But over several weeks this would be dangerous to the general health of the patient. The diet therefore represents a reasonable compromise between the nutritional needs of the individual and the speed with which the ultimate result needs to be attained.

Every physician I know that treats this problem is agreed that sugar is the most important item to be avoided. All sugars should be avoided, including cane sugar, beet sugar, powdered fructose, honey and maple (or any other) syrup.

I allow my patients to eat some fruits, which of course contain fructose, but restrict them to the fruits which contain the least amount, as shown in the diet below. Eating fruit rather than fructose is better as the fibre in the fruit slows the absorption of the fructose. Therefore, for most people I recommend the following diet (Phase 1) for 6 to 10 weeks depending on satisfactory progress.

Diet for treating the yeast syndrome

Phase 1

The following foods *only* to be eaten:

VEGETABLES

Artichokes (globe and Jerusalem)	Lettuce
Asparagus	Mange tout
Aubergines (eggplant)	Marrow
Avocado	Mung bean sprouts
Bamboo shoots	Okra (lady's fingers)
Bean sprouts	Olives
Black-eyed peas	Onion
Broccoli	Parsnips
Brussels sprouts	Peas – not petits pois
Carrots	Potatoes (baked, boiled
Cauliflower	or microwaved)
Celeriac	Pumpkin
Celery	Radish
Chick-peas	Red and green peppers
Chicory	Runner beans
Chinese leaves	Salsify
Courgettes (zucchini)	Soya beans
Cucumber	Shallots
Curly kale	Spices
French beans	Spinach
Garlic	Split peas
Ginger	Spring greens
Herbs (all fresh or dried)	Swede
Kelp (seaweed)	Tomatoes

Kohl rabi   Water chestnuts
Leek   Watercress

FRUITS
Only those on this list:
Guava   Lime
Honeydew melon   Rhubarb
Lemon   Watermelon

ALL MEATS
Including:
Beef   Pork
Chicken   Rabbit
Duck   Turkey
Lamb   Veal
Pheasant and all game birds   Venison
Offal (liver, kidneys, etc)
from any source

ALL FISH
(*NOT* breaded or battered) including:
Cod   Salmon (fresh and tinned)
Haddock   Sardines (fresh and tinned)
Hake   Sea bass
Halibut   Sole
Herrings (and kippers)   Trout
Mackerel (fresh and smoked)   Tuna (fresh and tinned)
Monkfish   Turbot
Plaice

ALL SHELLFISH
Including:

Crab

Crayfish

Lobster

Mussels

Oysters

Prawns

Scallops

Shrimps

Whelks

Winkles

DAIRY
Only those on this list:

Butter

Cottage cheese

Cream

Whole cows' milk
(in small quantities)

Edam cheese

Goats' milk

Gouda cheese

Soya milk

Yoghurt – *live* goats' or
cows' milk

DRINKS
No alcoholic drinks

Coffee

Black (ordinary) tea

Carrot juice (bottled or fresh)

Diet Cola and other diet sodas

Goats' milk

Green tea

Herbal teas

Soya milk

Tomato juice (bottled or fresh)

Water

MISCELLANEOUS

Basmati rice

Brown rice (wholegrain)

Oils – all cooking and salad oils

Rice cakes (organic)

Rice pasta

Seeds e.g. sunflower, sesame

Tabasco sauce

Tahini

Tofu

Once there has been some improvement, which should usually occur within about eight to 12 weeks, you can then expand your dietary repertoire into the Phase 2 anti-yeast syndrome diet.

Phase 2

To be followed for at least 10 weeks. The following foods to be added to those in Phase 1:

GRAINS

Barley

Buckwheat

Oats

Dried beans and pulses

Sweetcorn

Rye

Wholemeal wheat (soda bread can be made with bicarbonate of soda)

FRUIT

Only in small quantities:

Apples

Blackberries

Cherries

Gooseberries

Peaches

Pineapple

Pomegranate

Satsumas

Strawberries

NUTS

Only in small quantities:

Almonds

Chestnuts

Filberts

Hazelnuts

Peanuts

Most people continue to improve on this diet, and in a further two to three months they can expand into Phase 3, which returns the diet to almost normal, with the notable exception of the sugar products.

Phase 3

Phase 3 should be followed for 10 weeks. It may now be possible for you to introduce some yeast-related foods into your diet. To test your sensitivity to yeast, take three brewer's yeast tablets and note any adverse reactions that may occur over the next two days. If no adverse reaction occurs you may introduce into your diet the following items *that are to be taken in moderation.*

Cheeses (all types)	Vinegar
Mushrooms	Wholemeal bread
Gin	With low-calorie
Scotch whisky	mixers if wished
Vodka	
Dry wine (red or white)	

You can also introduce:

All other fruits	Pecans
Brazil nuts	Pistachios
Cashew nuts	Walnuts
Coconut (unsweetened)	

Plus you can add any other foods *not* containing sugar (dextrose / glucose / sucrose / fructose) or honey. *Be very careful* to look at all labels on every pre-packaged food product you buy. As long as you are well, sugar is allowed at times in small quantities, and if you do not see a return of the original problems (in which case all sugar consumption must stop), you are advised to keep your sugar consumption low, pretty well for the rest of your life.

Low sugar consumption means indulging in a few sauces, curries and maybe occasional confectionary, but no major return to added sugar in tea or coffee, cakes, biscuits etc. With the ever-increasing evidence that sugar is involved in a whole host of other major human illnesses, such as coronary artery disease (see Professor John Yudkin's book entitled *Pure White and Deadly*, published by Penguin, 1988) sugar restriction is pretty good advice for anyone interested in their health.

Specific medications for the yeast syndrome

Nystatin

The most effective medication for treating the yeast syndrome is nystatin. Nystatin has been used by doctors for over 60 years and has an enviable safety record. This safety record is partly because, except at very high dosage, it is not absorbed at all from the gut. In other words, it does not reach the bloodstream but remains inside the digestive tract, where it does all its work killing the yeast/fungi/germs situated within.

An illustration of the safety of this medication comes from the cancer institutes in America where some children were found to be suffering from virulent intestinal candidiasis as a result of the cytotoxic drugs that they had been given. Doses of 100 tablets a day or more of nystatin were used to treat those conditions and were found to be perfectly well tolerated. Nystatin is arguably the safest medication in the *British Pharmacopoeia*.

Most of the doctors I know use pure nystatin powder rather than nystatin tablets, which are obtainable at the chemist. I use pure nystatin powder because:

- it is much cheaper than the tablets which, when the full dosage is obtained, can be prohibitively expensive;
- the yeast organisms colonise the whole digestive tract from the mouth to the rectum, and, of course, tablets which are swallowed will not treat the organisms in the mouth or in the oesophagus;
- the tablets contain food colourings and other chemicals and filling agents, such as cornflour – these can contribute to the

food sensitivity problem or compromise an elimination diet;
- worst of all, the tablets are sugar-coated which somewhat defeats adhering to a sugar-free diet.

The nystatin powder must be stored in a refrigerator, but not in the freezer compartment. Although it is an extremely safe medication and has been used for over 60 years it is still a prescription-only medicine and as such has to be obtained from a doctor, such as many of my colleagues from the British Society of Ecological Medicine.

When I ran my clinic (The Burghwood) in Banstead, Surrey, I was able to supply our patients with pure nystatin powder and empty gelatin capsules. Most found it quite easy, all be it a bit fiddly, to fill the capsules themselves. Dr Pouria, who now runs the clinic (and who has written the Foreword to this book), still supplies the powder and capsules. Once filled, the capsules should be initially taken at a dose of one capsule twice daily, eventually building up, at five-day intervals, to 10 capsules daily. If you are prescribed nystatin by a doctor who is a member of the British Society of Ecological Medicine (see www.ecomed.org.uk) you will be given specific instructions about taking it. If you are prescribed it by your GP or other doctor who is not so familiar with treating the yeast syndrome I have included the detailed instructions in appendix II.

The Herxheimer response (die-off reaction)

The Herxheimer response is the name given to certain problems that can occur with some people as the dose of nystatin is increased. The problems do not occur only with nystatin but can occur with any medication that is effectively killing yeast/fungal organisms. The more effective the medication, the more likely the problem is to occur.

As the dosage of nystatin is increased, some individuals may at a certain dosage level notice a sudden increase in the severity of the very symptoms they are treating. Sometimes, in addition, headache, fatigue, depression and flu-like symptoms may also make an appearance. The symptoms are almost certainly caused by a sudden large increase in the production of yeast toxins. Nystatin kills yeast germs quite brutally, and in laboratory tests it can be shown that the cell walls of yeast cells disintegrate, releasing the yeast toxin held within. Consequently, if large quantities of yeast are killed there is a large release of yeast toxin in the digestive tract. Yeast toxin is absorbed from the digestive tract into the bloodstream and can lead to symptoms in any part of the body.

When the dosage of nystatin is lowered by about half a teaspoon, the symptoms will usually die away in three or four days. After another week or two of nystatin treatment at the slightly reduced dosage the individual will then usually be able to tolerate the dosage which previously produced the Herxheimer response, as more of the yeast germs have now been eliminated.

This response is named after Dr Herxheimer who, in the early part of the 20th century, described a similar response when patients were being successfully treated for syphilis. In the cases he observed, the syphilitic lesions could be shown to regress but the patient often started to experience joint pains and fever because of the toxin released by the dead spirochetes (syphilis germs).

Anyone experiencing this type of response can be virtually certain that they have a yeast problem, as people without the yeast problem have no trouble at all in taking any reasonable dose of nystatin. I have always thought that obvious Herxheimer responses are probably the single most positive diagnostic indicator of the yeast problem.

There are some people, it must be said, who have a great deal of trouble getting on at all with nystatin. These are usually those who look pale and ill, with multiple food and chemical sensitivities. They can have decidedly adverse reactions to even micro-doses of nystatin and usually need, at least initially, to be treated with small doses of something like caprylic acid or *Lactobacillus acidophilus* (see pages 118-9). There are a few people who will even have Herxheimer reactions to these milder regimes and who need to be treated with diet only, for a month or two, before active treatment can be initiated. Various manoeuvers can be tried in such people to get them through the early stages of effective anti-yeast/fungal treatment:

- *Candida* neutralisation. The technique entails finding a neutralising level of *Candida albicans* in the same way as other neutralisation therapy (see chapter 6). The person then takes daily subcutaneous injections of *Candida* extract, which can produce a considerable immediate symptom improvement, and seems to counteract the Herxheimer reaction. In some people, however, the neutralising level is rather unstable and has to be adjusted frequently.
- Temporarily (for about 10-14 days) eliminate all carbohydrate from the diet, while rapidly increased doses of nystatin are taken, and in these circumstances the doses can be well tolerated.
- Colonic wash-outs to eliminate excess yeast from the colon where they are usually at their most prolific.

Amphoterecin–B

This is an anti-fungal antibiotic which has a mode of action identical to that of nystatin. Like nystatin, it is not absorbed from the gut in the dosage we recommend. Data from many sources indicate that this drug is a safe alternative to nystatin and can be valuable (a) to those who cannot tolerate nystatin; (b) to those having a poor clinical response to nystatin; (c) to those who symptomatically relapse while taking nystatin, despite an initial apparent improvement.

Amphoterecin-B is currently available in the UK and is retailed under the trade name of Fungilin in 100 mg tablets. I usually try to work up to the maximum dosage suggested by the makers, which is two 100 mg tablets four times a day.

In hospital practice, amphoterecin-B is sometimes given by intravenous injection. Giving it this way is very effective in treating *Candida* in deeper tissues but is, however, decidedly dangerous as there is a risk of kidney damage. I would only advocate the tablet form of the medication, which is almost totally safe.

Fluconazole (brand name, Diflucan)

Fluconazole is a potent systemic anti-fungal drug. In contrast to nystatin and amphoterecin-B, this is absorbed from the gut and does get into the bloodstream, and from there to all parts of the body. Considering that it is distributed throughout the body, it is a remarkably safe drug and the only queries concerning its safety relate to people who are severely ill already, with conditions such as Aids and cancer. Except in such people, there is no suggestion of side-effects in the liver, kidney or other organs, and it has now totally replaced ketoconazole (Nizoral) in my affections.

Occasionally I did use ketoconazole in the past when it looked as if a systemic antifungicide would be invaluable, but one had to frequently monitor liver function (in particular, by blood test) as there is a well-documented risk (of less than one in 10,000) of severe hepatitis with this drug.

There are certainly people who seem to need a systemic antifungicide (that is, one that affects all parts of the body) over and above the intra-lumenal anti-fungals (those that are not absorbed beyond the inside of the digestive tract), such as nystatin and amphoterecin-B. I see the role of nystatin and amphoterecin-B being to reduce the gut reservoir and hence the source of the infection, and that of fluconazole as being to finish off the job by eradicating problems in the tissues once the gut reservoir is low. Certainly, clinically we have often seen major further improvement with fluconazole over and above that which we have obtained with nystatin.

I give fluconazole in a dosage of one 150 mg capsule a day for six weeks at the most. Fluconazole has been on the market for many years and its safety for long courses has been established. Professor Sydney Baker of the Gesell Institute in America has reported using the 200 mg capsules over the same time span with improved results in many people. However, it would be very rare for anyone who has a weight problem only, to need fluconazole.

Itraconazole (brand name, Sporanox)

Itraconazole comes in a 100 mg capsule and is a similar drug to fluconazole in that it is absorbed from the gut and distributed throughout the system. Like fluconazole, no serious side effects have been reported.

Obtaining anti-fungal prescription-only medications

Nystatin, amphoterecin–B, fluconazole and itraconazole are available only on prescription. Nystatin, which is the most useful medication, is often difficult for general practitioners to source in the powder form which is necessary. A good place to look to find a doctor that specialises in this problem is the British Society for Ecological Medicine (see appendix II).

My philosophy on drug usage

Some people who have read my earlier books may express surprise at my advocacy of these powerful drugs, so I think I should clarify my position at this point.

- I am against using drugs that exist purely to suppress symptoms without attacking the cause of those symptoms. Hence I dislike the use of anti-inflammatory drugs, painkillers, steroids, tranquilisers and so forth. I agree with the 19th century physician Constantine Hering who used to teach his students that the suppression of acute symptoms tends to cause chronic symptoms. I accept, however, that there are times when the use of these drugs in desperate circumstances may be justified.

- I am all for the use of drugs which get at the cause of the illnesses when this is possible. If I should contract meningococcal meningitis I would be taking penicillin as fast as I could lay my hands on it. Without it I would be dead in 24 hours; with it I wouldn't. If I get tuberculosis I will be the first in the queue for streptomycin and other potent anti-tuberculosis drugs. Most severe yeast-type problems would not get better within a reasonable time span, in my experience, without potent anti-fungals. They get at the cause of the problem and they are wonderfully safe.

Caprylic acid

This anti-fungal medication is a 'short-chain fatty acid', originally discovered over 30 years ago by Dr Irene Neuhauser of the University of Illinois. The recent huge upsurge in interest in yeast problems prompted various companies to dig up old research on anti-fungal substances, and this particular medication has proved to very useful. Caprylic acid is now retailed under various different names, but my current favourite is Mycopryl 400 (made by Biocare), which seems to work especially well because it becomes uniformly dispersed on the gut wall along the entire length of the intestine. The ultimate therapeutic dose is three capsules of Mycopryl 400 three times daily with meals, but as with other anti-fungals the dose has to be gradually increased, probably from three capsules a day slowly to nine over a period of about three weeks. If the capsules are taken just before meals this maximises the anti-fungal effect and minimises the belching which sometimes occurs after ingesting the capsules.

As caprylic acid is extremely safe it is retailed as a food supplement, and hence it can be bought over the counter at health food shops and is often advocated by naturopaths, chiropractors, and similar, unlike nystatin amphoterecin-B, fluconazole and itraconazole, which are only available on a doctor's prescription. The manufacturers of Mycopryl 400 suggest that its value may be enhanced if a high yield *Lactobacillus acidophilus* preparation is given at the same time. As with any other product that kills *Candida* effectively, it can lead to the Herxheimer or die-off reaction, and as with the other medications, the problem can usually be solved by temporarily reducing the dosage and then gradually increasing it again after more of the yeast cells have been eradicated. It is noticeable that the Herxheimer reactions with this product tend to be milder and less frequent.

Lactobacillus acidophilus

Lactobacillus acidophilus is a non-chemical approach to the yeast problem. It is a micro-organism which normally resides in the digestive tract of all people. On average, an adult will have approximately two and a half pounds of various micro-organisms present in the lower small intestine and colon. *Lactobacillus acidophilus* figures prominently in this proportion of micro-organisms and is wholly beneficial. There are over 200 known strains of it. My current preference is Bio-Acidophilus (made by Biocare), which contains the human strain of *Lactobacillus acidophilus*, as opposed to the cow (bovine) strain. The human strain is also in the Lamberts' product called Super Acidophilus Plus. It is considered that the human strain will probably survive much better within the human gut than the bovine strain. This is because the conditions of high acidity and high pancreatic enzymes present in the human gut are quite different from those found in the cow's gut, and the human strain of the *Lactobacillus acidophilus* will survive much better for these reasons.

Lactobacillus acidophilus exerts its beneficial influence by actively competing for space on the mucous membranes of the digestive tract with colonies of yeast/fungi. It is also thought to have a specific antagonistic effect on the yeasts. In general I find *Lactobacillus acidophilus* works far more slowly and less dramatically than nystatin or amphoterecin-B. Its main use, therefore, is in instances where the more potent drugs cannot be tolerated. It also aids beneficial recolonisation of the gut after the yeasts have been largely eliminated.

Garlic

This foodstuff has been used for medical purposes for centuries. Many scientific papers have now been published on the effects observed in the laboratory of garlic on strains of *Candida albicans*. One study, for example, showed that 24 out of 26 strains of *Candida albicans* were sensitive to aqueous dilutions of garlic extract. No large-scale controlled clinical trials of garlic have ever been conducted or are likely to be. The cost of such trials would be huge and if they strongly support the efficacy of garlic as an anti-fungal agent, who is going to make any substantial money out of retailing a substance that cannot be patented? This is a dreadful but mostly true comment on factors that influence medical progress.

Eminent physicians who have studied garlic state that it is a highly effective anti-fungal agent. Amounts small enough not to make your breath smell will have beneficial effects. The major chemical constituent of whole garlic which gives it its therapeutic effectiveness is allicin, which is also unfortunately responsible for the odour. Removing the allicin to remove the odour will also remove the anti-fungal effect. Garlic powder and whole garlic cloves are undoubtedly effective, but there is a distinct question mark in my mind as to the effectiveness of the odourless preparations.

Caprylic acid, *Lactobacillus acidophilus,* and garlic powder are freely available over the counter at good health shops.

Summary of medications

There is currently a great deal of discussion as to the various merits and demerits of the anti-fungal substances I have just described. In general, treatment of *Candida* has fallen into two distinct camps. On one side are the allopathic physicians who are legally entitled to prescribe anti-fungal medications such as nystatin and amphoterecin-B. These physicians also employ diets similar to the ones I described earlier in this chapter. A different route is followed by alternative health therapists such as chiropractors and naturopaths, who are legally unable to prescribe these drugs. They rely on caprylic acid, *Lactobacillus acidophilus,* garlic, oleic acid and biotin. In common with other allopathic physicians I do, however, make quite a lot of use of the more natural anti-fungal medications in people who are particularly sensitive to the Herxheimer-type response.

Clinical trials of nystatin and sugar-free/yeast-free diets

There have been no specific studies showing that treatment for the yeast syndrome can have a dramatic effect on weight problems, although every doctor I have known who treats this syndrome has observed marked weight reductions that are usually permanent.

Some people may think that it is the low carbohydrate content of the diet that is producing the beneficial response and not the anti-fungal medications. However, I have seen many people who have been on the diet for a while with no medication, showing little or no response. In contrast, the introduction of nystatin has, within two or three weeks, produced quite marked weight losses while the diet remained the same.

There have been studies showing very positive outcomes of this regime treating several conditions, especially psoriasis, urticaria, irritable bowel syndrome, recurring cystitis and recurring vaginitis.

There are various books on this subject, including *The Yeast Syndrome* by Dr John Trowbridge, and *The Yeast Connection* by Dr William J Crook. Dr Crook's book was top of the New York best seller list for over two months. Dr Orion Truss wrote the book *The Missing Diagnosis*, which started many doctors on exploring this avenue.

Case History – Julie H

Julie originally saw me with severe weight problems which she had had, to some extent, since she was four years old. She weighed 19 stone 5 lb (271 lb or 123 kg) and was 5 feet 10 inches (1.48 m) tall and aged 38. She was also suffering from severe arthritis and chronic fatigue easily leading to total exhaustion. Her history revealed a number of indications of food sensitivity, and she also had virtually all of the symptoms suggestive of a yeast problem mentioned earlier in this chapter. I decided to treat the food sensitivity first. After seven days on my elimination diet her joints had improved by 90%, her fatigue had gone completely and she had lost 12 lb (5.5 kg) in weight. She subsequently reacted to about six foods, and was able to discontinue all of the drugs she had previously been obliged to take.

In the next six months she lost a total of 6 stone 2 lb (86 lb or 39 kg), but plateaued at 13 stone 3 lb (185 lb or 84 kg). Although delighted by the impressive weight loss she felt she had more weight to lose and the symptoms of the yeast syndrome were still present. Accordingly, I put her on Phase 1 of the diet I have outlined in this chapter plus increasing doses of nystatin. Immediately her weight started to fall again and within the next three months she had got down to 11 stone 11 lb (165 lb or 75 kg). She had, therefore, lost a total of 7 stone 8 lb (106 lb or 48 kg) and all of her symptoms in just one year and three months without any quantity restriction in her diet. At her height (remember, 5 foot 10 inches (1.48 m)) she was more than happy with her final weight. She brought a track suit she used to wear when weighing nearly 20 stone to show me, and then delighted in showing how she could now get both of her legs into just one leg of the track suit.

When I saw her a year later she still weighed well under 12 stone.

Chapter summary

- I have frequently found that people whose weight problem is not caused by food sensitivity, respond very well to a yeast-free/sugar-free diet combined with anti-yeast medications.
- Yeasts such as *Candida albicans* (thrush) can exist in a yeast form, which is circular, or a fungal form, which has long thread-like extensions called mycelia. The fungal form is thought to be the one that causes most of the problem.
- At one time the yeast *Candida albicans* (thrush) was thought to be the precise cause of the problem, but it is likely that other yeasts are also involved.
- The gut fermentation test, as its name suggests, measures fermentation in the gut. It does so by estimating the quantity of ethanol (alcohol) produced after exposure to glucose. It is, in fact, a very good test for the yeast syndrome. After adequate treatment the excess ethanol disappears.
- The presence of certain symptoms (see page 102) makes the diagnosis more likely.
- The presence of various predisposing factors for yeast

overgrowth also makes the diagnosis more likely (see page 102).

- There is a questionnaire in chapter 14 which you should complete if you think you might be suffering from this problem.
- The condition is partially treated using a relatively strict sugar-free diet for two months (Phase 1) which expands to include more foods as you improve (Phases 2 and 3).
- Various anti-fungal medications are used in the treatment of this syndrome – some are prescription only and some are available over the counter. Those that are prescription only are nystatin, amphoterecin and fluconazole.
- This treatment has been 'road tested' in my clinic since 1982, with gratifying results.
- There are details in appendix III of how to take nystatin in the most effective way. The dosage described is as used by doctors who regularly treat this problem.

Chapter 8

Hypothyroidism as a cause of weight problems

'Hypothyroidism' is a common disorder in which the amount of hormone secreted by the thyroid gland is inadequate to meet the body's needs. This hormone plays a major part in the body's metabolism and if not enough is produced the body slows down. One consequence of this is often excess weight.

Many authors who write books on the management of weight problems mention hypothyroidism, as an obvious cause of weight problems, and I think this would not be disputed. However, they usually go on to say that conventional thyroid function tests are perfectly adequate, and if low output from the thyroid gland is suspected as a problem it can be identified by the appropriate blood tests, and treated with thyroxine (a synthetic thyroid hormone replacement). How wonderful it would be if it were that simple.

In this discussion I am not going to discuss hyperthyroidism (too much thyroid output), as this normally leads to weight loss and is consequently not relevant to this book.

Diagnosing hypothyroidism

Common symptoms associated with hypothyroidism are:
- increasing weight
- fatigue
- constipation

- general weakness
- thinning hair and loss of the outer third of the eyebrows
- cold hands and feet
- dry rough skin
- swelling around the ankles which does not indent (pit) with finger pressure.

Only rarely do all of these symptoms occur in one patient. Medical textbooks list up to 36 different symptoms that can occur but the above are the most common. Even these symptoms can be confused with food sensitivity or the yeast syndrome.

'How can I assess if I might have hypothyroidism?'

The physician, Dr Broda Barnes, was the first to introduce the early morning temperature test. You can either take your temperature by putting the thermometer under your tongue or in your armpit when you first wake up. This should be done before you get out of bed. It is necessary to leave the thermometer in place for at least five minutes. If you put the thermometer under your tongue then readings consistently lower than 36.6° C (97.8° F) might indeed indicate that you could have a problem with low thyroid. If using the armpit, problems may be indicated with readings lower than 36.0° C (96.8° F).

Many years ago, while I was visiting the USA, the prominent American specialist on thyroid function, Dr Howard Hagglund, told me a good physical indicator is the size of the little finger, and surprisingly I have often found this to be true. Place your hand flat on the table and look to see how far the little finger extends. Many people with hypothyroidism will notice that their little finger does not reach as far as the knuckle below the nail on the adjacent finger. Why this is the case is a complete mystery to me.

If you think there may be a possibility that you have a problem with your thyroid gland you need to see your doctor.

'What signs will my doctor look for?'

When your doctor examines you, s/he will be looking for:

- general hair loss, most significantly the outer third of your eyebrows
- a soft difficult-to-feel pulse
- cold dry skin
- a little finger shorter than normal
- a distinct swelling of the thyroid gland (a goitre).

If s/he suspects that you do indeed have a problem with your thyroid, s/he will most likely send you for blood tests.

Blood tests for hypothyroidism

Blood tests are, in my opinion a total nightmare. They are, to this day, steadfastly adhered to by most of the medical profession, though Dr Hagglund, has stated: 'Never be fooled by a normal thyroid blood test – it never was any good and never will be.'

Blood tests are taken to measure the component elements that the thyroid gland produces – namely T_1, T_2, T_3, T_4. These terms are short for very long chemical names. The most important ones are T_3 and T_4. The other critical test performed is to measure thyroid stimulating hormone (TSH) which is produced by the pituitary gland. Many doctors consider the test for TSH as the most indicative, as a raised level of this points to the fact that the thyroid is not responding normally.

Many doctors state that a normal TSH rules out hypothyroidism. What I, and many others in my profession, are absolutely sure about is that this simplistic view leads to misdiagnosis of large numbers of patients and condemns them to a life of misery, and lots of totally inappropriate drugs.

A lady medical colleague of mine had suffered for many years, with considerable weight gain, fatigue, cold extremities and hair loss. She had consulted an endocrinologist (a specialist in this field) as she suspected herself that she had hypothyroidism. He ordered all the usual blood tests, but they all returned absolutely within the normal ranges. He informed her that her thyroid gland was perfectly normal.

She later found herself sitting next to a friend of mine while listening to a lecture. This other doctor had an interest in this field and he told her that, in his opinion, blood tests do not pick up cases of hypothyroidism in about half of all cases.

At his suggestion she kept a record of early morning temperatures which only reaffirmed her original suspicions of hypothyroidism. She also sent a 24-hour urine sample (see below) to a major European laboratory near Antwerp. They tested her urine levels for T_3, T_4 and TSH. In her case the level of T_3 was low but her T_4 was normal. He then treated her with natural thyroid extracts.

The great disadvantage of any blood test is that it only measures what is going on at one moment of time, the moment when the blood was taken. Thyroid hormones are released in pulses (short spurts) and so three blood tests taken in three subsequent hours may give widely differing results. An alternative to a blood test is a 24-hour urine test. This test involves collecting all the urine that you pass in a 24-hour period and by doing so it evens out any fluctuations in the output of all thyroid hormones.

When I next saw her six months later I almost didn't recognise her, as she had lost over two stones in weight and looked 10 years younger. In addition she was much brighter and her whole demeanour had changed.

In my own clinic I had seen several patients who had been told that their thyroid gland was normal on the basis of normal blood tests. T_3 is the hormone that does the 'business'. The inability to convert from T_4 to T_3 is the usual problem in difficult-to-treat genuinely hypothyroid patients, and giving such patients ordinary thyroxine tablets (T_4) doesn't help them at all. I accordingly referred them to Thyroid UK who could put them in touch with specialists who understand the problem in their area.

In May 2000 the *British Medical Journal*[19] published an article by Denis St John O'Reilly, a Consultant Clinical Biochemist in the Department of Thyroid Disease at Glasgow Royal Infirmary. The article was titled 'Thyroid Function Tests – time for a reassessment'.

He pointed out that in the year 1999, one in six of Scotland's 5.1 million population were tested for TSH. In the UK as a whole, the figure was one in 10. He stated that a remarkable downgrading of the clinical aspects of hypothyroidism had paralleled the inexorable increase in the number of thyroid function tested performed in the preceding 20 years. This had led to chaos in the diagnosis of hypothyroidism. Some of the most salient points in this long clinical paper were:

- There are no data on the relative importance of biochemical thyroid function tests and clinical symptoms and signs in assessing poor thyroid function.
- The secretion of TSH is influenced by many factors other than the feedback from the thyroid gland.
- One study involving 1580 hospital inpatients found that blood thyroid function tests showed abnormal results in 33% of patients tested.
- Ninety per cent of these abnormal test results were later found to be wrong in that they diagnosed thyroid disease when it didn't exist.

However, this trend has continued unabated since this paper. This is partly due, in my view, to the tendency to move towards laboratory-based medicine rather than assessing the patient as a whole person.

At the end of the day I strongly advise anyone NOT to attempt self-treatment with hormones obtained from the internet. Such hormones are very powerful drugs and can be extremely dangerous. They therefore must have medical supervision. If you suspect you have a thyroid problem you should see your GP. If you are not happy with your conventional treatment then you could contact either Thyroid UK or the British Society for Ecological Medicine who can put you in touch with doctors who use a different approach. I also recommend you get hold of a copy of Dr Barry Durrant-Peatfield's guide to the subject, based on many years of treating patients with this problem: *Your Thyroid and How to Keep it Healthy.*

The cholesterol myth and why low-fat diets are a major cause of weight gain

How do we know low-fat diets make weight problems worse?

There is a vast quantity of medical literature describing the consequences of the change to low-fat diets. One very eloquent example was published in the *British Medical Journal* in 1995, detailing findings from the Medical Research Council. This reported that between 1980 and 1991 the number of people in the UK who were overweight doubled. If you think about it, this is an extraordinary fact by itself. In 11 years you might expect, possibly, a small percentage increase, but for it to double is remarkable, particularly when you remember that it took decades to reach the first level. It becomes even more extraordinary when you learn that in those same 11 years the average total calorie intake in this country fell by 20%. Approximately the same thing happened in the USA at about the same time. This is described in chapter 10.

So perhaps everyone had given up on exercise? Again, the answer is a resounding 'no'. Between 1970 and today there has been a vast and progressive expansion in the exercise industry, with the opening of countless gyms and fitness centres, accompanied by the publication of innumerable exercise DVDs. In the

1950s, women in particular did not indulge in this sort of activity, yet were much slimmer. In 1980 the *Washington Post* announced 100 million Americans were now involved in the new fitness revolution. It also said that a decade earlier they would all have been described as 'health nuts'.

The revolution on both sides of the Atlantic was obviously prompted by the rapid increase in weight that many were observing. So, in the UK from 1980 to 1991 people in general exercised more and ate 20% fewer calories yet obesity rates doubled. It is hard to comprehend, yet this trend is continuing to get worse right up to today. By far the biggest dietary change from the late 1970s was the adoption of low-fat diets, linked to the 'cholesterol theory'. Low-fat diets are, in my opinion, a major cause of obesity. As they follow the recommendations of the medical profession in general, it is important for me to explain why they are not healthy and should not be adopted. This chapter and chapters 10-12 are dedicated to this end.

Low-fat diets are used extensively in many countries but especially in the USA, Mexico and Great Britain. They are used for two reasons:

- Fats are the foods which have the highest density of calories and therefore would be a logical item to reduce if one believes in low-calorie diets; remember my reasons for describing them as being worse than useless in chapter 2?
- Fats are regarded as dangerous foods to eat because of the fat (cholesterol) heart theory originally proposed by Dr Ancel Keys in the USA.

In the USA, the cholesterol heart theory is regarded by many citizens as certain as night follows day. In many other countries doctors and patients are rather more sceptical. In America, the consumption of fat is currently the lowest per person in the world yet the Americans have the distinction of being the fattest nation. In the late 1970s American people were told by the American Heart Association and other public health bodies to reduce fat strictly, and eat more carbohydrates, even refined ones. Since that gem of advice was given just before 1980 the epidemic of obesity in the USA has increased from 13% in 1980 to 33% by 2006.

The Mexicans are the second fattest nation on earth; they are rather influenced by their richer neighbours. The UK is third and the worst part of the UK is Scotland. In 1951 the average adult woman in the UK wore size 12 clothes, but by 2005 the average size had increased to 16. In England in 2009, 24% of men and 25% of women were officially classified as clinically obese. The number of people who were just 'overweight' was 42% of men and 32% of women. As in the USA, the rate of increase has been growing in the last two or three decades. Thus the proportion of the population in the UK who are overweight is now similar to the USA. When it comes to full-blown obesity as opposed to merely having weight problems the USA is way ahead, at a third of the entire adult population.

By way of contrast the French eat the most fat[20] of all types and French women are the slimmest of all nations in Europe. French men are the third slimmest, making the French as a nation the slimmest in Europe. The French diet is loaded with saturated fat in the form of butter, cheese, cream, eggs, liver, meat and rich pates.

In the USA the average consumption of sugar is around 168 lb (76 kg) per person per year. In the UK it is approximately 144 lb (65.5 kg) per person per year. In France it is only 50 lb (22.5 kg) per person per year.

Not only are the French the slimmest nation in Europe but they also have a very low rate of coronary artery disease.[20] In the USA, 315 out of every 100,000 middle-aged men die of heart disease every year, whereas in France the rate is 145 out of every 100,000. In the Gascony region of France where goose and duck liver form a staple part of the diet, the rate is even lower at only an amazing 80 deaths per 100,000 per year.

If the French could reduce their cigarette consumption, which is quite high, their coronary artery disease rate would probably be even lower. These figures are not disputed but are just described as the French paradox and ignored by the 'cholesterol establishment' in the USA and UK. Yet this is in effect a huge ongoing clinical study comparing statistics from two similar western industrial societies. One is France with a population of around 50 million and another is the USA with a population 320 million. This must be extremely clinically significant because of the large numbers involved.

Forgetting statistics, one has only to walk around a French provincial town, where there are few British or American tourists, to observe lots of slim French women and men. The opposite occurs in the USA and UK and particularly in some parts of the USA.

Switzerland has the second highest consumption of fats[21] in Europe and again has low incidences of obesity and coronary artery disease. The Italians have noted the French experience and their women are virtually as slim as the French. So we now have the Swiss and Italian paradoxes to add to the French one!

In Spain we find yet another paradox. In 1995, using national statistics, researchers in Spain found[22] that between 1964 and 1991 consumption fell of:
- bread by 53%,
- rice by 35%,
- potatoes by 53%.

During the same period consumption rose of:
- beef by 96%,
- pork by a massive 382%,
- poultry by 312%,
- full cream milk by 73%.

Obviously the Spanish took a dim view of the cholesterol theory. So did this cause an increase in heart disease? The short answer is, no. In this particular period heart disease deaths fell by 25% in men and 34% in women.[22] High blood pressure rates also fell, and death by strokes also decreased.

So now we have the French, Swiss, Italian and Spanish paradoxes!

Finally, many people have heard about the Mediterranean diet, particularly that eaten in Crete in 1960 (this was when the coronary rate reached its highest). In Crete the rate per 100,000 of deaths from coronary artery disease was a remarkable 10 deaths only per year.[23] At the time it was thought that this was attributable to a diet high in vegetables and olive oil, but such a diet was eaten in many other places whose statistics were not nearly so impressive. The statistics available initially did not differentiate between refined and unrefined carbohydrates. What we now know is that the Cretans only consumed 16 lb (7.5 kg) of sugar per person per year, and they ate wholemeal bread virtually exclusively.

I have much more evidence to offer to you later in this chapter that is highly suggestive that the cholesterol theory, on which promotion of a low-fat/high-carbohydrate diet is based, is the main reason for the obesity epidemics in North America and the UK. It is, in fact, the vast increase in consumption of sugar and other refined carbohydrates, caused mostly by the emphasis on fat restriction, which is primarily responsible for this increase in obesity.

The role of food in human evolution

Although this is a book about weight problems, the problems of weight, diabetes and coronary artery disease are very closely interconnected and I have found it impossible to address weight alone as what causes one usually causes the others as it were. To understand how these problems have developed over many years we need to understand how the food we eat has gradually changed us.

It is now commonly accepted that there have been five major developments in the human diet:

- At the very beginning, around six million years ago, we were initially purely vegetarian.
- The change to a nomadic Stone Age diet that included meat and animal products occurred at around 2.3 million years ago.
- The use of fire for cooking 800,000 years ago led to a radical change in what we ate. By being able to make meat and vegetable matter more easily digestible we no longer had to eat large quantities of raw food.
- The change from being nomadic hunter/gatherers to a more settled way of life occurred around 10,000 years ago when we started growing grains.
- The introduction of refined carbohydrates and processed foods started around 1850 and gathered momentum until the present day.

Our original hominid ancestor, called *Australopithecus*, appeared around six millions years ago and was the first to start walking upright. S/He was purely vegetarian and had a small brain and large abdomen like the apes. The large abdomen was needed for the diet of fruit, nuts and vegetables, because these had to be consumed in large quantities to provide enough nutrients. *Australopithecus's* successor, approximately 2.3 million years ago, was called *Homo habilis* (or 'Handyman'). S/He had learned to use crude tools, usually stones which allowed for butchery. It has been noted that the skull and brain of Handyman were larger than those of *Australopithecus*. The tools allowed her/him to cut into the carcasses of dead animals and smash bones to remove the marrow. S/He seems initially just to have been a scavenger but eventually learned to hunt alongside still gathering fruits, nuts and vegetables. We have, therefore, as a species eaten meat for some 2.3 million years.

Chapter 9

The first truly human form, *Homo erectus*, appeared 1.8 million years ago. S/He was characterised by having a very much enlarged brain, but much smaller abdomen than previously. His/her increased brain power enabled him/her to co-operate with others and thus hunt in groups. As *Homo erectus*, in general, was not able to run as fast as most animals, it is thought that s/he succeeded by using devices such as snares.

Later, somewhere around 800,000 years ago, our ancestors found they could use fire to cook their food, and that meat and vegetables tasted better and were easier to digest. Cooking is, in fact, a predigestive mechanism thus requiring less energy to digest, thereby leaving more energy available for other essential survival mechanisms.

As the human brain gradually became larger, the abdomen was becoming smaller. It is generally agreed that the development of the human brain was entirely a result of the consumption of meat, and in particular, fat. The human brain has defined what it is to be human and has allowed our species to dominate this planet despite our relatively puny physical status. Thus we have eaten saturated fat for 2.3 million years, during which time it has been not only beneficial to our development in general, but absolutely critical to the development of our advanced brain and higher intellect.

Without meat and the marrow from bones our ancestors would not have been able to move out of Africa and to colonise the colder northern areas of Europe. In the winter months, if they had been dependent on finding plant food, they would have starved to death. The palaeoanthropologist, Mike Richards of Oxford University, studied the bones of Palaeolithic people who inhabited England around 12,000 years ago. He found that their diet was almost identical to that of top-level carnivores, such as wolves and bears.

There then occurred the first 'agricultural revolution' when the planting of wheat, corn and other grains occurred, originally in Egypt and other countries in that region. This allowed our species to become more settled in one area and lessened its reliance on its hunter/gatherer activities.

Cereal grains initially had a lot of adverse health effects, as any major change in diet has on any species. One indication of this was that the average height decreased dramatically. The average height of a man fell from 5' 9" to 5' 3" while the average height of women fell from 5' 5" to 5' 0". Bone diseases like osteoporosis, rickets and dental cavities became more common, while life expectancy reduced. Despite the initial adverse effects of a diet rich in cereal grains, right up to the mid-19th century there was still little obesity, no diabetes and no coronary artery disease.

Only in 1912 did we have the first recorded appearance of coronary artery disease, yet we are now being told to believe that animal fat has become a major health hazard.

Along came refined carbohydrates

Around 1850 came the initial production of refined carbohydrates, such as refined sugars, white flour and white rice. White flour was made by separating the outer layers of the grain, containing fibre, and virtually all the vitamins and proteins, from the starch. The starch is composed of long chains of glucose molecules.

Refined white sugar is made by removing the juice containing sucrose from the surrounding cells and husk of the cane sugar plant or beet sugar plant. In both cases the more refined the product the lower the vitamin, mineral, protein and fibre content. The same is true of white rice, which has been through a similar process to wheat.

These refined grains soon led to huge epidemics of B vitamin deficiency disorders, such as pellagra and beri beri, all around the world. For example, a major epidemic of pellagra occurred between 1906 and 1940 in the southern states of America, killing over 100,000 people and affecting three million. It was caused by a deficiency of the B vitamin called niacin (B_3) and the amino acid tryptophan, both problems being common in people eating refined corn at that time. In south-east Asia, beri beri was caused by a deficiency of another B vitamin, thiamine (B_1), which happened when people changed to eating white instead of brown rice. Like pellagra, it ceased to be a problem when the appropriate B vitamins were added back into these foods.

Only in the past 30 years has the amino acid, homocysteine, been found to play a significant part in coronary artery disease. This condition is again caused by a much more subtle but long-term deficiency of B vitamins, in this case B_6 (found in whole grains, especially wheat germ), B_{12} (found in meat and dairy products), and folate, or 'folic acid' (B_9). I will discuss this further in chapter 11.

To return to the topic of refined sugar, it was originally a luxury until the mid-19th century, when it came to be grown throughout the western world as either sugar cane or sugar beet.

In 1874, tariffs on sugar importation were removed and sugar consumption rapidly increased from very little to more than 90 lb (41 kg) per person per year in the UK by 1900. Similarly, the Americans had reached 80 lb (36 kg) per head per annum by the start of the First World War.

So when did the coronary artery disease epidemic begin?

The first medical reports of coronary artery disease in the UK are not too clear. Certainly the first doctor to publish a clinical paper on the condition was Dr James Herrick,[25] a Chicago physician, in 1912. However, by 1920 coronary artery disease was still rare in America and when Dr Paul Dudley-White introduced the German electro-cardiograph to his colleagues at Harvard University they were not very interested as the condition for which it could be used was so rare. This new machine could identify the presence of arterial blockages in the coronary arteries of the heart, allowing the early diagnosis of coronary artery disease. These days every cardiologist and many GPs still use this machine in a somewhat more advanced form.

Dr Dudley-White had to search for patients who would benefit from his new technology but during the next 40 years the incidence of this disease rose dramatically, so much so that by 1970 it was causing 40% of all American and British deaths. Dr Dudley-White went on to become President Eisenhower's cardiologist when he had his first coronary thrombosis. This did much to increase awareness of the condition worldwide. The idea that coronary artery disease was rare before the 1920s was confirmed by many famous physicians of the day.

So this condition started probably, at the earliest, around 1905 as it is quite possible that the first few cases were missed.

In the early 1900s British Royal Navy surgeon, Captain Thomas Latimore ('Peter') Cleave spent many years studying the effect of refined carbohydrates when they were first introduced to native populations previously unexposed to such food. As a result of this work he introduced his rule of a 20-year time lapse between the first introduction of these foods and the serious complications that can follow. This same rule applies to cigarette smoking, for example, which takes at least 20 years to start causing serious adverse effects. Probably a consumption of 70 lb (32 kg) of sugar per head per annum in any population would be enough to trigger incidences of diabetes after approximately 20 years' consumption. This level of consumption was probably reached by some Americans and Britons by around 1885. If we add 20 years to this date it would neatly fit in with the commencement of coronary artery disease around 1905-10 in the US. It was probably at least as prevalent in the UK at this time, but it is very difficult to obtain any statistics.

During these same years the consumption of animal fats was dropping in the US due to the huge increase in the American population, as a result of mass immigration, and the failure of the livestock industry to keep pace with the growing demand. Putting it another way and through a slightly different time frame, in the 60-year period from 1910 to 1970 the proportion of traditional animal fat in the American diet reduced from 83% to 62%. Butter consumption plummeted from 18 lb (8 kg) per person per year to just 4 lb (<2 kg). During the same period the percentage of dietary vegetable oil in the form of margarine, shortening and refined oils increased 400%. Finally, the consumption of sugars and processed foods increased about 60%.

Dr Ancel Keys, the main proponent of the cholesterol theory, claimed there had been an increase in the consumption of animal fats in the 20 years prior to the first appearance of coronary artery disease. The statistics show this was totally fictitious as there was a marked decrease. Thus the first appearance of coronary artery disease followed a period of significant reduction in animal fat consumption combined with a signficant increase in refined carbohydrate consumption. The cholesterol theory that eating too much saturated fat gives us heart disease does not fit the facts at all.

The missionary doctors

The 'missionary doctors' were physicians who went to various remote parts of the world to practise medicine and were in a position to observe the impact on their patients of refined carbohydrates, when these were introduced to a previously whole-food diet. The World Health Organisation (WHO) originated the term 'nutrition transition' to describe this process. White flour, white rice and white sugar were the commonest items to be sent to these various primitive peoples. The white flour and rice were particularly popular as during their journey to these countries these products were not attacked by rats and beetles. I maintain if the rats and beetles don't want them, then neither do I!

Sir Robert McCarrison later convinced the authorities in Great

Britain to add specific B vitamins to white flour which lessened some of the worst effects of this foodstuff.

Two of the earliest missionary physicians were, Capt. 'Peter' Cleave as mentioned already, and Dr George Campbell. Peter Cleave spent most of his medical career with primitive peoples around the Singapore region. He knew of Dr Campbell who started his medical career as a GP in Natal (South Africa). Dr Campbell focused mainly on Indian immigrants living in Natal and the local Zulu population in the early parts of the 20th century. He observed that the local European population suffered from obesity, diabetes, hypertension and coronary artery disease. The rural Zulus and Indian immigrants did not suffer any of these complaints. Later he spent a year working at the University of Pennsylvania. The African-American population there were suffering the same diseases as the Europeans in Natal. He later returned to Natal. After some years had passed and the nutrition transition phase had occurred, he became particularly interested in diabetes, and found a large difference between the sugar-cane cutters whom he noticed virtually never developed diabetes and the other patients who were now eating refined sugar. The cane sugar cutters were getting their sugar in the unrefined form straight from the plantations.

Unrefined sugar absorbs very slowly in contrast to refined sugars that absorb rapidly into the bloodstream. The 'non white' people now eating refined sugar frequently developed obesity, diabetes and coronary artery diseases at levels previously only seen in the Europeans. Campbell considered they would need to eat more than 70 lb (32 kg) of refined sugar per annum for between 18 and 22 years to develop diabetes, and a further 20 years or so to develop coronary thrombosis. Obesity was seen to start very much earlier. In the early 1960s he corresponded frequently with Capt. Cleave and in 1966 they published a book called *Diabetes, Coronary Thrombosis and the Saccharine Disease*, 'saccharine' meaning, in this case, related to sugar. In this book they argued that diabetes, coronary artery disease and obesity were primarily related to refined sugar.

To cut a very long story short, their findings would explain why the same diseases would appear after the arrival of refined carbohydrates in peoples who previously had existed exclusively on unrefined whole foods. Other investigators had studied other indigenous peoples with similar findings, including the Inuit Indians (Eskimos) of Northern Canada and Alaska, the Masai of Kenya, the Sanboro nomads of Kenya, the Aborigines of Australia and the North American Indians of the Great Plains.

Capt. Cleave wrote that the refining of carbohydrates represented the most dramatic change in human nutrition since the introduction of agriculture. There is no chance of us as yet being adapted to this concentration of carbohydrates as these products have only been around for just over 160 years, which in terms of evolution is not even yesterday.

This concentration of carbohydrates by refining, leads to over consumption in three ways:

- By reducing the volume it is much easier to eat more. Capt. Cleave contrasted the eating of a teaspoon of sugar with the same amount of carbohydrate contained in an apple. A person can easily consume, say, seven teaspoons of sugar in the form of a carbonated beverage, but seven apples would be a completely different proposition.
- The refining process dramatically increases the rate of absorption and the onrush of blood sugar to the pancreas and the subsequent release of large quantities of insulin.
- As I pointed out in chapter 4, refined sugar is a common food allergen, and being sensitive to a food can lead to cravings for it, which in turn leads to over-consumption.

In 1977, Capt. Cleave was asked to attend a meeting of a committee set up in the USA to take views from physicians known to hold differing opinions on the validity or otherwise, of the cholesterol theory. It was chaired by Senator George McGovern. Capt. Cleave first confirmed his belief that coronary artery disease was due entirely to the consumption of refined carbohydrates. He said, 'I don't hold the cholesterol view for one moment,' stating that mankind had been eating saturated fats for hundreds of thousands of years with no sign of coronary artery disease.

He said, 'For a modern disease to be related to an old-fashioned food is one of the most ludicrous things I have ever heard in my life. If anybody tells me that eating fat was the cause of coronary artery disease I should look at them in amazement. When it comes to those dreadful sweet things that are served up, that is a very different proposition.'

John Yudkin, Professor of Nutrition at Queen Elizabeth College, London, England (see page 144), totally agreed and personally blamed refined sugar entirely for heart disease. He was equally adamant that neither saturated fat nor cholesterol played any part at all. Later work showed that Capt. Cleave was right in that both refined sugar and white flour were a major cause of coronary artery disease (see chapter 11).

How then did the cholesterol theory originate in the first place?

The cholesterol theory actually started in the mid-19th century, although at that time there were no clinical cases of coronary artery disease reported in journals. Rudolf Virchow, a pathologist working in Berlin, noticed when he worked on human autopsies that the arteries in the bodies he examined often showed thickening and plaque formation.

He found that on microscopic examination these plaques contained cholesterol. No one was interested at the time as it was over 60 years later that the first cases of coronary artery disease were recorded. Around 50 years after Virchow's work Russian scientist Nikolai Anitschkov[24] force fed rabbits a high animal-fat diet. Their arteries thickened and filled with cholesterol. However, rabbits are exclusively vegan and feeding such animals pure animal fat when they have no biological mechanism for dealing with it is quite absurd. In no way could these results mimic the human experience. Scientists were rightly highly critical of these findings which they mockingly referred to as the 'cholesterol disease of rabbits'.

Anitschkov took on board these criticisms and agreed that the experiment had no practical significance for humans. He then performed similar experiments on dogs, rats and humans. These experiments showed there were no increases in blood cholesterol and hardening of the arteries in these other naturally fat-eating species. Although deeply flawed, his original work with rabbits did sow the seed of the new theory that coronary artery disease might have something to do with cholesterol. Strangely his later work never found its way into the medical textbooks.

In the 1950s it was discovered that oxidised cholesterol components called oxycholesterols produced injury to arterial walls with deposition of plaques containing cholesterol when fed to rabbits and monkeys. At that time Albany Medical College showed that highly purified cholesterol freed of all traces of oxycholesterols and protected from the oxygen in the air does not produce arteriosclerosis at all, even when given to rabbits or monkeys. As Anitschkov and Von Virchow did not have the technology to do this purification or prevent contamination all they had managed to show was that oxycholesterol contaminants could produce arteriosclerosis, but nothing about cholesterol itself.

After the cholesterol theory had been proposed it was logical to set up studies looking for evidence that a population of patients would benefit from a low-fat diet compared with a population eating a normal diet for their country. There were three studies, which I will discuss in the next section, that appeared initially to show some positive support for the cholesterol theory but which over time showed something very different.

In the rest of this chapter I will demonstrate that the consumption of saturated fats or other naturally occurring fats has nothing to do with obesity, diabetes and coronary artery disease. I consider the main reason for the epidemic of obesity in the UK and USA to be the huge and increasing consumption of refined carbohydrates and the limitation of fat consumption.

Research looking at dietary fats and heart disease

The Seven Countries study by Dr Ancel Keys

The cholesterol theory proposes that coronary artery disease, which was first reported in 1912 and had reached epidemic proportions by the 1970s, resulted from the consumption of fats, principally saturated fats, especially cholesterol. High consumption would result in high levels of cholesterol in the blood, and over time in fatty plaques forming in the arteries – especially the arteries that feed the heart – until those arteries would become so constricted they could easily be blocked by a blood clot (thrombosis).

Dr Keys was, without doubt, the prime mover in the development of this theory. His first major contribution to it was the Seven Countries study in 1970.[23] This appeared to show that countries that had high saturated fat consumption had high death rates from coronary artery disease. This was immediately criticised on the grounds that those countries whose statistics he chose were those that would neatly fit his case. They were:

- Finland
- USA
- Italy
- The Netherlands
- The former Yugoslavia
- Japan
- Crete.

At that time there were 15 other countries which had amassed adequate statistics and when these results were added to the original seven there was no significant correlation between saturated fat consumption and coronary artery disease.

The Framingham heart study

The Framingham heart study started in 1948 and involved 6000 people living in a small town called Framingham in Massachusetts. It had already become famous as it had successfully proved cigarette smoking was the major cause of lung cancer and a major contributor to coronary artery disease. There were plenty of other studies with similar findings, including the famous study on British doctors authored by Sir Richard Doll and Sir Austin Bradford-Hill.

In the early days of the Framingham study Dr Thomas Dawber, who led it, announced that cholesterol levels in the blood were a definite risk factor for coronary artery disease. He had found that the risk of heart disease for those Framingham men whose cholesterol level had been over 260 mg per dl was five times greater than it was for men whose cholesterol had been below 200 mg per dl. This was initially considered one of the most significant pieces of evidence that Dr Ancel Keys hypothesis was correct. In fact, this became the most important piece of evidence for this theory. By 1971, however, as the men from Framingham aged, those who died of heart disease became ever more likely to have low cholesterol levels, rather than high. The theory that high cholesterol might lead to heart disease in women was tenuous under the age of 50 and non-existent for women older than 50. By 1971 the Framingham investigators noted that cholesterol levels had no predictive value at all. Thus the Framingham Study no longer supported the cholesterol theory. From initially being one of the greatest supporters of the cholesterol theory, it became one of its greatest critics. These later results were never published in any medical journal.

Dr George Mann (of whom more later) who left the study in the 1960s recalled that the National Institute of Health (USA) refused to allow publication of the results. In my opinion it is indefensible that the National Institute of Health, which is supported entirely by public funding, blocked this vital information from being made public.

The Helsinki mental hospital study[31]

The third of the studies that did initially show some positive support for the cholesterol theory was the Helsinki mental hospital study. What was studied was not a low-fat diet but a high-polyunsaturated/low-saturated fat diet. The study ran between 1959 and 1966 and appeared to reduce heart disease deaths by a half. However, when all causes of death were taken into account the male low-fat dieters seemed to live only marginally longer, and female low-fat dieters had no benefit at all. It was decided to continue this study for a further 10 years. After this period, the low-fat dieters who were in the original study then became twice as likely to die of heart disease as those in the control group who ate normally.

Summary of original evidence

So, the Seven Country study, the Framingham study and the Helsinki study were all hailed as good evidence for the cholesterol theory in the early days, but eventually proved to be the contrary.

Subsequent studies on heart disease

I will now identify and summarise the four largest studies ever published exploring the relationship between saturated fat consumption and coronary artery disease. They are:
- Women's health initiative study[26] USA involving over 48,000 women
- Malmo (Sweden) study[27] of over 28,000 people

- The Minnesota (USA) survey[28] involving over 9000 people
- The MR-FIT (Multiple Risk Factor Intervention Trial)[29,30] USA which screened over 360,000 men for serum cholesterol, then studied the 3.33% (12,000 men) who had the highest cholesterol readings.

The women's health initiative study[26] USA was reported in 2006, having lasted for 8.1 years. The treatment group increased their consumption of fruit and vegetables to five servings daily while the control group ate what they felt like. By year six of the diet, the treatment group were consuming 29% of calories as fat but in the control group fat was 37% of calories. The result of this trial showed that there was no significant difference in the incidence of coronary artery disease or death between the two groups. There was also no difference in the incidence of strokes, or death from strokes. The incidence of cancer and death from cancer were also the same for both groups. This study cost a staggering $400,000,000.

The Malmo (Sweden) study,[27] published in 2005, involved over 28,000 middle-aged men and women. This trial was split into four categories from low to high saturated-fat intake. The follow-up was undertaken six and a half years later. This study concluded that the consumption of saturated-fat did not have any effect on cardiovascular disease or mortality in men. However, in women, there was actually a lower incidence of death from cardiovascular disease with increasing saturated fat consumption. The conclusion of this study was reported as: 'This study does not support the concept that saturated fat causes coronary artery disease.'

The Minnesota coronary survey[28] was performed at the University of Minnesota's Department of Nutrition from 1968 to 1973, and included over 9000 men and women in six state mental hospitals. The group that were studied were all on a diet low in saturated fat and dietary cholesterol. The control group, again, were eating as they liked. The average serum cholesterol level dropped by 15% for those on the low-cholesterol diet. Although their cholesterol levels were 'successfully' lowered, there was an increased rate of heart disease in this group. Altogether, 260 people in the cholesterol-lowering diet group died of coronary thrombosis compared to only 206 in the control group.

At first this study was not published at all. (I wonder why?) It was finally published by Dr Frantz 16 years later (a year after he retired) in a little-read journal called *Arterial Sclerosis*. When asked by Gary Taubes, the eminent scientific journalist, for the reason for the long delay in publication, Dr Frantz replied: 'We were just disappointed in the way it came out.'

The timing of the publication of this Minnesota coronary survey[28] was of critical importance. It was completed by 1974 and was the biggest study in the USA at that time. It showed a conclusive increase in death from heart disease in people on a low-saturated-fat diet. Between 1974 and 1978 there was extensive debate on the validity of the cholesterol theory, but the Minnesota study had been kept from prying eyes. It is inconceivable that the McGovern Committee could have recommended a diet low in saturated fat for the entire American nation had they been aware of the results of this study. By the time it was finally published in the academic backwater of a little-read journal, the die had been cast. A real tragedy.

Gary Taubes has written a phenomenal book, which is well worth reading, called *The Diet Delusion,* going into great detail concerning how the population at large has been constantly misinformed about the role of fat in heart disease.

The MR-FIT study[29,30] followed just the 3.33% of men who had the highest serum cholesterol reading out of the original 360,000 who were screened. These 12,000 were divided into two groups with one half following a low-cholesterol diet and the other eating what they wanted. On the low-cholesterol diet, the consumption of cholesterol was reduced by 42% and saturated-fat consumption by 28%. This study lasted for seven years, with the results being published in 1982. There was found to be no difference in the incidence of heart disease between the groups. The difference in the death rate between the groups was negligible, but was actually slightly higher in the group following the low-cholesterol diet.

Thus these four studies, involving nearly 100,000 people, all clearly demonstrated no benefit, whatsoever, from eating a low-fat diet. In fact two of the studies revealed increased, not decreased, cardiac death on a low-fat diet.

When there are several studies all basically looking at the same field of interest, scientists from all backgrounds use what is called a meta-analysis to establish the collective results. This is really a study of studies. Those studies included in the meta-analysis must meet certain criteria so as to ensure they are comparing like with like.

The Cochrane Collaboration was set up to carry out such meta-analyses. In 2001 it published a review of trials that studied the effect of reduced fat or modified fat consumption in the treatment of cardiovascular disease. It concluded that these studies showed no effect on longevity and no significant effect on cardiovascular disease. In 2006 it published a further report, which was a review of multiple risk studies. These studies looked at the effect of different factors on cardiovascular health, including eating fat/cholesterol and lowering blood pressure. It identified 10 really good studies. The pooled results from all these studies showed, even by attempting to correct multiple risk factors, no significant effect on mortality was achieved.

In 1988, the Surgeon General of the USA decided to collect all the evidence linking saturated fat to heart disease. It was said this would be the definitive study, coming from an impeccable source. (This, incidentally, was how the Framingham study was described when its initial findings seemed to support the saturated fat causes heart disease concept.) However, 11 years later this study was aborted. To explain the somewhat surprising turn of events a letter was circulated that: 'The Office did not fully anticipate the magnitude of the additional expertise and staff resources that were needed.' It would be interesting to surmise what the investigators had been doing for 11 years when references to approximately 30 studies could be obtained within a few days. Eventually Dr Bill Harlan of the Oversight Committee and associate director of the Office of Disease Prevention at the National Institute of Health commented: 'The report was initiated with a preconceived opinion of the conclusion; however, the science behind those opinions was clearly not holding up. Clearly the thoughts of yesterday were not going to serve us very well.'

This could probably be translated as: 'We couldn't find anything to support the fact that saturated fat in the diet caused heart disease.' In a nutshell, after many years and the expenditure of countless millions of dollars, they chose not to publish their findings as they did not support their preconceived ideas. Unhappily they chose to say nothing, because they probably preferred not to upset their colleagues in the cholesterol community rather than inform the American public and the world at large of the real truth.

Cholesterol is an essential nutrient

Our livers manufacture 80-90% of the cholesterol in our blood stream to ensure we have adequate supplies for all the many and various functions for which we need it. In fact, the fat that our livers produce is almost entirely saturated. It is unlikey that our livers would produce saturated fat if it were dangerous for us.

Cholesterol is needed for many important functions:

- Growing babies need to consume their mothers' milk, which contains a higher proportion of cholesterol than is found in any other food. This milk also contains over 50% of its calories as fat, much of it as saturated fat. These fats are essential for the proper growth of babies, especially in the development of the brain. Even so, the American Heart Association is now recommending a low-cholesterol/low-fat diet for children. Most commercial brands of formula milk are low in saturated fats and some are almost devoid of cholesterol. Have the American Heart Association gone completely mad? It is such incredible arrogance to suggest that mother's milk contains dangerous ingredients and that a group of doctors know better than nature. This could well help create obesity at even younger ages.

- Cholesterol is needed for the production of brain synapses which are essential connections between nerve cells in the brain. These synapses are made almost entirely from cholesterol.
- Cholesterol is the raw material for the production of almost all sex hormones. These hormones are an essential part of good health.
- Vitamin D is synthesised from cholesterol, by the action of sunlight. Deficiency of this vitamin is a known contributor to breast cancer and this fact partly explains the lower incidence of breast cancer in Mediterranean countries where there is, of course, more sunlight.
- Cholesterol is a key component of bile, the substance that is released from the gall bladder via the bile duct into the small intestine, where it is vital for digestion.
- Every cell in our bodies uses cholesterol as a key structural component of the cell membrane. Without cholesterol cells would disintegrate and the membrane function would be severely disrupted.

Changing opinions

Dr Kilmer McCully wrote in his book, *The Homocysteine Revolution*, that: 'It is significant that the 80 year history of the cholesterol approach has yet to provide a coherent and comprehensive scientific explanation which explains in detail how cholesterol, a normal constituent of the body, or excess dietary fat in the diet of susceptible populations, produces atherosclerotic plaques [as in coronary artery disease – author].' Before he became totally disillusioned with the cholesterol theory, on which he had worked for many years, Dr McCully was a leading researcher at Harvard Medical School.

Even Dr Ancel Keyes, the main protagonist of the cholesterol theory, eventually stated in 1997: 'There is no connection whatsoever between cholesterol in food and cholesterol in the blood, and we have known this all along. Cholesterol in the diet does not matter at all unless you happen to be a chicken or a rabbit.'

In 1998, Dr William Castelli, then Director of the Framingham study (see page 147), said: 'The more saturated fat one ate, the more cholesterol one ate, the lower the person's serum cholesterol. We also found that people who ate the most cholesterol and ate the most calories weighed the least and were the most physically active.' This observation, of course, explains the French 'paradox' statistics. The French eat large amounts of fat yet have a low rate of coronary artery disease, and are also slim. Here we can see vividly illustrated the fact that cholesterol levels in the blood might have some value as a risk factor for possible disease, but in no way represent a cause of disease. In other words, consuming fat in any form, whether it be saturated fat, or unsaturated fat, has no adverse effect on heart disease or weight problems. Thus, this study, which initially was the greatest supporter of the cholesterol theory, became one of its greatest critics.

Dr George Mann, who was an earlier Director of the Framingham Study, stated: 'The diet/heart hypothesis has been repeatedly shown to be wrong, and yet for complicated reasons of pride, profit and prejudice the hypothesis continues to be exploited by scientists' fund-raising enterprises, food companies and even governmental agencies. The public is being deceived by the greatest health scam of the century.'

In defence of butter

No discussion of this subject would be complete without a mention of margarine vs butter. Margarine has outsold butter by a considerable margin in the UK and USA for a long time. It must be pointed out that margarine is an entirely man-made food, and has no similarity to any fat found in nature. The problem with liquid fats like the various vegetable oils is that they are liquid at room temperature and therefore difficult to spread on bread or bake with.

Hydrogenation is the process that turns polyunsaturated fats into a fat that is solid at room temperature. The manufacturers start with one of the cheapest oils such as corn or soya bean oil. This oil is then mixed with tiny metal particles, usually nickel oxide, which is very toxic when absorbed by the body. It is impossible to totally eliminate this from the final product. The oil with its nickel catalyst is then subjected to hydrogenation. This is achieved in a high-pressure and high-temperature reactor where the oil is bombarded with hydrogen atoms.

Soap-like substances and starch are then squeezed into the mixture to give it a better consistency. The product is then again subjected to high temperatures when it is steam cleaned to remove its offensive odour. At this point the margarine's appearance is still that of an unappetising grey sludge. Coal tar dyes and strong flavours must then be added to make it resemble butter. Sounds wonderful, doesn't it?

The process of hydrogenation leads to the formation of transform (often just referred to as 'trans') fatty acids which are very toxic, and the human body does not recognise them. Instead of being eliminated, as are naturally occurring fatty acids, they become incorporated into the body's cell membranes. In turn, this causes your own cells to become hydrogenated. Once in place these altered fats block the utilisation of essential fatty acids. These margarines may have contributed in the past to the increased mortality often seen with low-cholesterol diets.

In contrast, butter is a completely natural product that has been eaten for very many years. The body is able to deal with it effectively. Because it is a saturated fat it is not damaged by high temperatures such as those attained when frying. In my opinion it is still a healthier choice, even than those margarines that now no longer contain trans fats.

By 2011 the description 'margarine' had disappeared from British supermarket shelves due to the considerable disquiet among consumers at the presence of trans fats. Food manufacturers are now selling 'spreads'.

Statins

Statins were, like many drugs, discovered entirely by accident. A plant called 'red yeast rice' was discovered in a valley in Northern China by a researcher from the US government. As part of its defence mechanism this plant produces a poison known as lovastin to protect itself against its predators – herbivores – who will die should they eat it. Interestingly, this poison was found to block an enzyme called HMG Co A reductase. This enzyme facilitates an important step, amongst others, in the pathway of cholesterol synthesis in the liver. About 85% of cholesterol is manufactured by the liver with the body only obtaining around 15% from food sources. As I have already described, our livers produce so much cholesterol because it is so essential (see page 153).

Poisoning that vital pathway probably accounts for most of the side effects that these drugs have. However, statins do quite definitely lower serum cholesterol and they do reduce the risk of coronary thrombosis (blood clot). The main disadvantage, in a nutshell, is that virtually all of the statin drugs that show some reduction in death rates from coronary artery disease show an increase in death rate from other diseases, which at least partly cancel out the improved rates from heart disease.

My main worry about statins is the fact that in the USA pharmaceutical drugs can be advertised on TV, and frequently are. The only other country in the world that allows this is New Zealand. As statins are particularly big selling drugs they are advertised continuously on American television. Many of these adverts claim that the drug's benefits arise from lowering cholesterol; as such, they reinforce the whole cholesterol/fat-is-bad idea. I have demonstrated throughout this chapter that low-cholesterol diets have no value in promoting health in any way and that the low consumption of fat is a major reason for the epidemic of obesity.

There is plenty of evidence to support the view that statins are beneficial in heart disease, but there is virtually no evidence that they do so by lowering cholesterol. The reasons for this are:

- Other specific cholesterol-reducing drugs have shown no benefit whatsoever.
- The benefit that people with pre-existing heart disease receive is apparently very quick, in fact much quicker than could be obtained by lowering cholesterol.
- The benefit occurs whatever the patients' original cholesterol levels were – that is, even if they were normal or low to begin with.
- Statins help to some extent with strokes, though cholesterol levels have never been directly related to strokes.
- There is some evidence that statins decrease fibrin which is an integral part of the clotting mechanism that causes thrombosis.

Several drug companies accept that the way statins work is a mystery. Various academics have put forward complex mechanisms. There is no doubt that statins do work even if we do not fully appreciate how, so if I had coronary artery disease I would certainly be prepared to take them. I would not, however, contemplate going on a low-cholesterol diet, or take statins just because my cholesterol level was raised.

Conclusion

Eating fat has nothing whatsoever to do with becoming fat, and nothing to do with diabetes or coronary artery disease. The concept that eating fat is bad for you and your health is the biggest mistake in medical thinking in the past century. So what does cause these problems? In fact all of these problems have everything to do with the consumption of refined carbohydrates. When refined carbohydrates are not consumed obesity is rare, and diabetes and coronary artery disease are non-existent. Which, incidentally, explains why diabetes didn't appear till around 1875, and coronary artery disease was not reported until 1912.

Chapter summary

- The human race consumed animal fat for 2.3 million years without any sign of cardiac problems or diabetes. During that period, our brains, which are largely composed of fat, progressively enlarged, and we became more efficient at hunting and gathering.
- Eventually, we became the dominant species on this planet, and our enlarged brains allowed us to develop into the advanced cultural and scientific beings that we are today.
- Approximately 10,000 years ago the first 'agricultural revolution' began, introducing grains into our diet. This allowed mankind to change from a nomadic lifestyle to a more settled one. We were then able to rely less on meat, vegetables, fruit and nuts. We still continued to eat lots of meat, especially during the winter months in the more northern areas.

- The next major dietary revolution was the introduction of refined carbohydrates, starting around the mid-1800s. These new foods were unique in that they were absorbed into the bloodstream very quickly, resulting in high levels of insulin. Eating these foods placed a considerable strain on the pancreas, a situation that had never before occurred in the entire history of mankind.

- Twenty years or so after the initial introduction of refined carbohydrates there was an increase in weight problems; 40 years later, diabetes was becoming more common; 60 years later, the first cases of coronary artery disease were reported.

- Meanwhile, during this period there was a reduction in the consumption of animal fats due mostly to the rise in consumption of refined carbohydrates. In the USA, mass immigration in the late 1800s made it impossible for the livestock industry to keep up with the rising demand.

- When coronary artery disease started to become a problem, the medical profession chose to blame a food (saturated animal fat) that had been eaten for millennia. They exonerated refined carbohydrates, the only recent major addition to the diet. If that wasn't crazy enough, these refined carbohydrates were then introduced to various primitive peoples around the world who had previously lived only off meat, fish and other whole foods.

- Within the next few decades all these primitive peoples developed the same sequence of health problems as the developed world, culminating in the arrival of coronary artery disease.

- Incredibly, paying no attention to these events, the medical profession became fixated on the concept that saturated animal fat, after more than two million years of remarkably good behaviour, had decided to attack us!

- Amongst the western industrial nations, France has the

highest consumption of fat, and the lowest consumption of carbohydrates (particularly sugar), but is the slimmest nation, and has a death rate from heart disease that is less than 40% of the UK's or USA's.

- There have been more than 30 major studies comparing populations on low saturated-fat/cholesterol diets with people eating normally. These have involved well over 100,000 people. Not one study has shown any improvement in the death rate from coronary artery disease amongst the low-fat dieters.

Chapter 10

How refined carbohydrates cause weight and health problems, and the role of low-carbohydrate diets

The object of dieting is to lose fat and only fat, not muscle. We use two primary sources of fuel for energy production, fats and carbohydrates. Each one has its own metabolic pathway. Normally we use both. However, if one pathway is not working efficiently, the body shifts towards the other pathway which will become more dominant.

The majority of people will, if limited to only 20 grams of carbohydrate per day, be forced to burn fat. This will lead them to produce ketones in their urine (see later in this chapter). A few will fail to do this, and these people will not easily produce ketones because they are not good fat burners. These people may need other strategies, which I will discuss in more detail later. Either way, the carbohydrate content of the diet needs to be reduced by one means or another.

The opposite of this happened in the late 1970s onwards when everyone was instead advised to restrict fat and pay less attention to restricting carbohydrates. This led to obesity rates doubling in the UK and USA in the next 10–11 years, and trebling by the year 2002.

So, restricting carbohydrates and especially refined carbohydrates plays a major part in some people's weight-loss strategies.

This applies particularly to people who are excessively over-weight with disordered pancreatic function caused by years of over-consumption of refined carbohydrates.

In 1862, William Banting became the first person (as far as we know) to be treated with a low-carbohydrate diet. He was a wealthy intelligent fashionable undertaker, but weighed 14 stone 6 lb (202 lb or 91.5 kg) and was only 5 feet 5 inches (1.65 m) tall. Being so overweight he had to walk downstairs backwards to avoid jarring his knees, and couldn't tie his own shoelaces. For years he went from one doctor to another but all failed, despite their reputations, to do anything to reduce his weight. He tried Turkish baths, spa treatments, violent exercise and drastic diets amongst many other approaches. Despite all of this he either gained weight or stayed the same.

Eventually he noticed that he had a mild problem with his hearing so he went to see an ENT surgeon, Dr William Harvey. Quite reasonably Dr Harvey observed that Banting's problem was obesity, not deafness. He suggested an entirely new type of diet – a low-carbohydrate one. In less than a year Banting had lost nearly 50 lb (22.5 kg) in weight and 12.5 inches (32 cm) from his waistline. Not only did he lose all of this excess weight, but he felt exceptionally well throughout the process.

By modern low-carbohydrate standards, his diet was very un-constrained and did contain small amounts of carbohydrate and a fair amount of various alcoholic beverages (spirits). In total he was consuming 2800 calories a day. Previously, on a diet restricting his calories to 1000 a day, he had lost no weight whatsoever. He said, 'I can now confidently say that the quantity of the diet may be safely left to the natural appetite and that it is the quality only that is needed to abate and cure corpulence.'

Dr Harvey, who designed the diet, had realised that it was carbohydrates (starch and sugar) that fattened most fat people.

In 1863 Banting self-published a 16-page pamphlet entitled: *A Letter on Corpulence Addressed to the Public*. This set off the first diet craze and his letter on corpulence sold very well throughout Europe and the USA. The craze went from strength to strength and within a year the word Banting had entered the English language as a verb meaning to diet. Many, including royalty, enthused over his diet, but the medical journals of the day were, predictably, less than complimentary. As a medical friend of mine says, 'the not-invented-here syndrome'.

General practitioners and many other doctors who were, however, happy to find anything that helped their patients with obesity, restricted carbohydrates either a lot or at least to some degree. Over the next hundred years many patients on this regime did well, and certainly better than those on the low-calorie, low-fat diets that became popular in the 1970s and which continue to the present day.

In the 1950s and the subsequent decade, obesity was not a major problem. In 1951 the average adult female in the UK wore size 12 clothes, but by 2008 the average size had become 16. The situation in the USA was even worse.

As I have already described, it was in the late 1970s that the cholesterol obsession really started to get a hold, mostly in the USA but also in the UK. The American Heart Association and other public bodies took it upon themselves to recommend stringent fat restriction and positively encouraged carbohydrate consumption – be it refined or unrefined. Americans in particular were terrified of becoming one of the 40% dying of coronary artery disease and so they concentrated on fat restriction. Weight reduction became less of a priority and this started the massive and unprecedented obesity explosion particularly affecting the USA, Mexico and the UK. Crazily, fat restriction was not only used as a treatment for 'the cholesterol problem', but also to achieve weight loss partly on the grounds that fat contained a high concentration of calories. This change has proved to be a total disaster and I have maintained for over 20 years that the cholesterol theory has been the main cause of the American and

British obesity epidemics by restricting fat while encouraging carbohydrate consumption.

It is bad enough to restrict fat, but it is much worse to increase refined carbohydrates at the same time. In the last quarter of a century, average Americans have been consuming 500 calories a day more than previously, and 90% of those calories are derived from carbohydrates (mostly refined). If someone asked me how he could become fatter I would tell him to eat as much refined carbohydrate as he could and carefully restrict fat in his diet.

Fats satiate appetite for many hours. In the absence of fat people rarely feel full and often resort to snacking. Snacks almost invariably consist of carbohydrates. Fat consumption puts the brakes on your appetite. Trying to diet with very little fat is like driving without brakes – that is, there is nothing to stop you. Without fat you need vast resources of willpower which the average person can't summon for long periods of time, as it makes life miserable. With plenty of fat in the diet this is not the case, so life in general becomes easier.

Low-carbohydrate diet books

The first British book discussing low-carbohydrate diets was written by John Yudkin, who was Professor of Nutrition at Queen Elizabeth College of Medicine in London. The book was called *The Slimming Business*. Yudkin in particular felt that sugar caused most of the problems being attributed to refined carbohydrates. He also, a little later, wrote another book called *Pure White and Deadly*, concentrating on his thesis that sugar was the primary cause of coronary artery disease, diabetes and obesity.

Dr Richard Mackarness, a few months later in 1957, published *Eat Fat and Grow Slim*, which I thought was a particularly good title for a book on low-carbohydrate diets. The gist of his book was that Stone Age man was very rarely fat and prior to the start of agriculture 10,000 years ago mankind ate meats, fish, fruits, nuts and vegetables. As a species we are not well adapted to cereal grains as we had spent six million years without them, prior to the birth of agriculture.

As stated earlier, in chapter 4, when Dr Mackarness was promoting his book *Eat Fat and Grow Slim* in Chicago a doctor said to him that his diet might work well because it avoided most of the common food sensitivities, such as cereal grains and sugars. This doctor told Dr Mackarness that his brother-in-law was Dr Theron Randolph who was famous in the USA for his work on food sensitivity and its role in many chronic illnesses. Meeting Dr Randolph led Dr Mackarness into a totally different direction, eventually culminating in his second book, *Not All in the Mind*, published in 1976. It was at this point that I became involved with Dr Mackarness and we remained close friends for over 20 years. Dr Mackarness and I confirmed that the low-carbohydrate diet theory was correct and important clinically. However, it worked for some people simply because it eliminated the foods to which they were sensitive. Other low-carbohydrate diet books include *Calories Don't Count* (1966), *The Doctors Quick Weight Loss Diet* (1968), *Dr Atkins' Diet Revolution* (1972) and onwards, *The Complete Scarsdale Medical Diet* (1978), *Protein Power* (1996), *Sugar Busters* (1998), *The Dukan Diet* (2000), *The Paleo Diet* (2002), *The South Beach Diet* (2003), and *Trick and Treat* (2008).

The Atkins diet went through a number of modifications, and became far and away the most famous diet book in history. Atkins deserves enormous praise for making his book exceptionally user-friendly, and sticking to his guns in the face of virulent opposition from the American Heart Association and the American Medical Association. This hostility occurred despite irrefutable evidence that low-carbohydrate diets had a genuine scientific basis and were completely safe.

Scientific validation for low-carbohydrate diets

The first study in 1957 was entitled 'A scientific evaluation of the Banting diet', authored by Professor Alan Kekwick and Dr G. L. Pawan[32] at the Middlesex Hospital in London. Obese people were admitted to hospital and were closely monitored while on the diet. The doctors proved that Banting was absolutely correct and concluded that the composition of the diet does indeed alter the expenditure of calories in obese patients: it increased when fat and proteins were eaten and decreased when carbohydrate was eaten. This work had a widespread effect on medical opinion when it was published, but most physicians have forgotten it since.

In the February 1957 edition of the *American Journal of Antibiotic Medicine and Clinical Therapy* it was stated that Professor Kekwick and Dr Pawan from the Middlesex Hospital in London reported good news for the obese. All the obese patients studied lost weight immediately after admission to hospital, and therefore a period of stabilisation was required before commencing investigation.

They found that if the proportion of fat, carbohydrate and protein consumed was kept constant, the rate of weight loss was proportional to the calorific intake. If, however, the calorific intake was kept constant at 1000 calories per day the most rapid weight loss was noted with the high-fat/high-protein diet. When the food intake was raised to 2600 calories, daily weight loss could still occur provided that this intake was eaten mainly in the form of fat and protein.

It was concluded that 30–50% of weight loss was derived from the total loss of body water and the remaining 50–70% from the loss of body fat.

In other words, this was a complete scientific validation for doctors basing weight control diets on carbohydrate restriction only. It also refutes the theory that when losing weight, a calorie is a calorie is a calorie wherever it comes from. It also contrasts with the loss of muscle mass seen on low-calorie diets.

Kekwick, Pawan and others also discovered that patients could still lose weight if they consumed up to 60 grams of carbohydrate daily in addition to fat and protein, but the weight loss was much greater if the carbohydrates were restricted to 20 grams, as in the induction phase of the Atkins diet.

Several other studies were performed to confirm Kekwick and Pawan's findings. One in 1965 was authored by Dr Frederick Benoit[33] and associates at Oakland Naval Hospital in the USA. They decided to compare the effects of a 1000 calorie high-fat diet that included 10 grams of carbohydrate with those of fasting. There were seven men in each group, all weighing between 230 and 290 lb (104.5–131.5 kg). On the 10-day fast there was a loss of 21 lb (9.5 kg) on average. Most of this weight loss was in lean body weight and only 7.5 lb (3.4 kg) was of body fat. However, on the high-fat-and-10-grams-of-carbohydrate diet, an average total loss of 14.5 lb (6.6 kg) was recorded. Of the 14.5 lb lost in weight, 14 lb was body fat. This confirms other studies showing a very high loss of subcutaneous fat on high-fat/high-protein diets. Thus, only 7.5 lb (3.4 kg) of body fat was lost on a total fast compared with 14.5 lb (6.6 kg) on a high-fat/high-protein diet.

In addition, the patients on the total fast lost a great deal of potassium, which can be quite dangerous for the heart, whereas those on the high-fat diet maintained their levels of potassium.

How eating refined carbohydrates causes major health problems

Diabetes

In the last 60 years there have been huge advances in our understanding of the metabolism of carbohydrates. These discoveries are very supportive of the value of low-carbohydrate diets. As time has passed the connection between obesity, type II diabetes and heart disease has become ever more obvious. The cause of diabetes in young people is a result of insulin deficiency. This occurs because of inefficient production by cells in the pancreas. This is known as insulin-dependent, or type I, diabetes. Type II in contrast is predominantly a disease of adults, linked to excess weight and insensitivity to insulin (they have enough insulin but are not responding to it).

Insulin is a hormone and it has the major role in regulating energy production, utilisation and storage. For many years it has been accepted that insulin's primary function is to remove sugar from the bloodstream and store it in the subcutaneous fat. The inability to do this is the main factor in the high levels of glucose found in the bloodstream and that signal diabetes. Insulin, in fact, has many roles including the regulation of fat, carbohydrate and protein metabolism. Thus it is involved with everything connected with the storage and use of all types of nutrients.

The rapidly increasing use of refined carbohydrates with their rapid absorbability and high concentrations of sugars presents a unique challenge to the pancreas and its production of insulin. This has never occurred before in the history of our evolution. Blood levels of glucose rise very rapidly after the digestion of refined carbohydrates and, in response, insulin levels rise equally rapidly. When this happens frequently blood levels of insulin become continuously raised, causing what doctors call 'hyperinsulinaemia' (too much insulin in the blood). Some of the glucose is converted to glycogen, a starch, which is stored in the muscles and liver. The rest is converted to triglycerides which are the main constituent of subcutaneous fat. Consequently, insulin is frequently referred to as the fat-producing hormone.

Until 1960 there was no way in which insulin in the blood could be accurately measured. Drs Yalow and Berson then discovered an accurate method, for which Dr Yalow was awarded the Nobel Prize for Medicine in 1977. They had shown that people who developed diabetes had very high levels of insulin in their bloodstream. Up to this time it had been assumed that diabetes was caused by low levels of insulin. Critically, it was the ability to measure insulin levels in the bloodstream that revolutionised the old view of diabetes. Of vast importance, obese patients were also found to have raised levels of insulin.

In 1965 these same doctors discovered an explanation for the contradiction that diabetics appeared to be lacking in insulin, but actually had high insulin levels, high blood sugar levels and sugar in their urine. This work led to the discovery of 'insulin resistance', in which ever larger amounts of insulin are needed to produce the normal response.

The next major step was the discovery that insulin resistance could actually be measured. The first test was published by Dr Reaven in 1970, but further improvements were made until the test had become completely reliable by 1980. Eventually, the American Diabetic Association became convinced that resistance to insulin was the fundamental defect in type II diabetes. The obvious consequence of all this was that refined carbohydrate should be restricted. This was quite definitely Dr Reaven's view. Soon after, he received the American Diabetic Association's Banting Medal for Scientific Achievement.[34]

Despite all this, the public health bodies in the USA refused to endorse the restriction of carbohydrates for any health reason whatsoever. Thus the science had been officially accepted, but the practical implementation of it had not. It's quite difficult to imagine what further sort of evidence would actually be needed to convince them. I don't think it could be scientific evidence as that already exists for the refined carbohydrate ⟶obesity ⟶diabetes ⟶heart disease concept.

The scientists mostly agreed that:
- Carbohydrates, especially refined ones, are the only food that stimulates the production of excess insulin.
- Insulin is known as the 'fattening hormone' as it is the only hormone leading to surplus storage of fat.

- Type II diabetics and people who are clinically obese both show high levels of insulin in their bloodstreams.
- Insulin creates its effect with the help of the enzyme lipoprotein lipase (LPL) as described in chapter 2. There is much more LPL activity after the consumption of refined carbohydrates.
- High levels of insulin in the blood eventually lead to insulin resistance and this in turn leads to even more insulin secretion.
- More and more fat is accumulated until the fat cells themselves become insulin resistant.
- Later still, exhausted pancreatic cells finally lose their ability to respond.

According to the NHS Information Service, diabetic drugs cost the NHS £725 million in 2010/11, an increase of 41% since 2005/6. There are now 2.5 million people in the UK with type II diabetes and, in addition, a further 850,000 are thought to have it, but are, as yet, undiagnosed. Over 33,000 people die from diabetes every year which makes it the fourth largest cause of death in the UK.

People with diabetes are, of course, at much greater risk of heart disease because, as I emphasise later, both conditions have similar causation. Other problems commonly found in people with type II diabetes are eyesight impairment and poor blood flow to the limbs leading, in extreme cases, to the need for amputation. The most common early symptoms are increased thirst with increased need for urination.

Now let me quickly summarise what we know about type II diabetes:

- It is initially suspected by finding sugar in the urine.
- The diagnosis is firmed up by finding a raised fasting blood sugar.
- It is completely confirmed by a glucose tolerance test (see page 172) that is positive.

- In the UK and USA the first few cases of type II diabetes occurred around 30 years after the initial production of refined sugar.
- When refined sugar is introduced to primitive people, type II diabetes starts to occur around 18-22 years later if they have been eating over 70 lb (32 kg) per year.
- For around 100 years doctors treated type II diabetes with strict restriction of sugar believing, not unreasonably, that it was caused by sugar consumption. The results were mostly effective.
- The biochemistry leading to the development of type II diabetes is as described already in this chapter.

There surely can be no doubt at all that refined sugar is the cause of type II diabetes.

Nowadays, would you believe, much of the current medical advice is entirely to stop talking about what causes diabetes and instead to concentrate on the treatment which they say should be:

- A low-fat diet because diabetics have a high risk of coronary artery disease. This is despite the fact there is not one single study showing low-cholesterol diets to be of any benefit in coronary artery disease let alone diabetes.
- They also suggest a high-carbohydrate diet despite the fact that it has been known for over a hundred years that refined sugar causes diabetes.

Have the patients finally taken over the asylum? This advice is absolute madness. Since these recommendations, the incidence of diabetes has exploded in line with the increase in obesity.

Coronary artery disease

Dr Reaven[35] measured both triglycerides and glucose tolerance in patients who had just suffered a coronary thrombosis (heart attack caused by a blood clot).

The glucose tolerance test has been used for many decades as the classic test for diabetes. After fasting overnight the patient's blood glucose level is measured. S/he is then given a high dose of glucose by mouth after which his/her blood glucose level is measured at half-hour intervals for the next two and a half hours. High blood sugar levels indicate that the patient has been unable to metabolise the glucose properly, and the problem is diagnosed as glucose sensitivity. This usually progresses to become diabetes.

Dr Reaven[35] reported that patients who had just had a coronary thrombosis ALWAYS had both high triglyceride levels and glucose sensitivity. The only common cause of both of these findings was insulin resistance, suggesting that insulin resistance was a probable cause of coronary thrombosis.

Thus these patients had what became known as 'carbohydrate induced lipaemia': in other words, high levels of fat in the blood as a result of eating refined carbohydrates. In these patients, blood fat levels increased when they ate refined carbohydrates and decreased when they ate fat. Although refined carbohydrates have been implicated before in coronary thrombosis, we know that we can exonerate whole grains because in the 10,000 years that they were eaten unrefined there was no diabetes or coronary artery disease.

Thus insulin resistance leads to both diabetes and heart disease and this can be summarised as shown in Figure 10.1.

This diagram will be expanded in the next chapter when I explain the role of chromium deficiency and vitamin B deficiencies, both of which are caused by the consumption of refined carbohydrates such as sugar and white flour.

Figure 10.1: How eating refined carbohydrates can lead to coronary artery disease

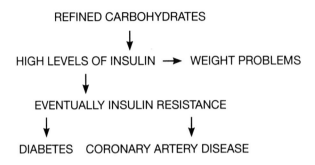

REFINED CARBOHYDRATES
↓
HIGH LEVELS OF INSULIN → WEIGHT PROBLEMS
↓
EVENTUALLY INSULIN RESISTANCE
↓   ↓
DIABETES   CORONARY ARTERY DISEASE

Working at Stanford University of Medicine, California, scientists in 2000 compared the effects of low-fat/high-carbohydrate diets[36] with high-fat/low-carbohydrate diets on blood cholesterol and triglyceride levels. The results of this study showed that people on the high-carbohydrate/low-fat diet had significantly higher blood triglyceride levels and significantly lower HDL (high-density lipoprotein). Both of these readings (high triglycerides and high HDL) are very adverse findings. This particular diet (high-carbohydrate/low-fat) is the diet that most Americans have been advised to follow. The authors concluded that given the dangerous potential of these changes it was appropriate to question the wisdom of recommending a low-fat/high-carbohydrate diet to all Americans.

In 2004 Dr Lars of the Ryden Karolinska University Hospital, in Sweden, confirmed Dr Reaven's finding of high glucose levels in patients with coronary thrombosis. He said: 'Forget cholesterol. The strongest predictor of a future heart attack was a high blood glucose.'

In 2001 another similar study showed that when blood glucose was raised for significant lengths of time the risk of heart attack was greatly increased.

These findings are so important because they do not describe what happens 10 years before or one year before a heart attack. They show what is happening at the time of the heart attack.

Raised blood insulin levels (hyperinsulinaemia)

In the early chapters of this book I explained that food sensitivity, an excess of yeast in the gut and hypothyroidism are major causes of weight problems. However, people who are dramatically overweight may have badly compromised the workings of their pancreas, and have perpetually high levels of insulin or full-blown insulin resistance. Such a person who has sorted out any food sensitivity or yeast syndrome problems may need to go onto a good low-carbohydrate diet if they are still overweight in order to rest their pancreas.

Blood tests indicating problems with carbohydrate metabolism

The following tests may be useful in assessing whether you should go onto a low-carbohydrate diet.

- **Plasma insulin levels** are very often raised in people with weight problems to a greater or lesser degree.
- A **glucose tolerance test** is also worth discussing with your physician. Obviously if it indicates diabetes you have a serious problem with carbohydrates. People showing a 'pre diabetic curve' are at risk too, as it is also a strong indicator of a misfiring carbohydrate metabolism.
- It is also worth considering asking for **serum cholesterol levels** and also **triglyceride levels**. Knowing these is useful for comparison when retesting several weeks into the diet. The cholesterol level should normally have reduced slightly and the triglyceride level dropped dramatically, confirming that these levels of serum fat are due to problems with carbohydrates. Certainly in trials of the Atkins diet triglyceride levels dropped dramatically.

Limited-carbohydrate diets

There are basically four types of limited-carbohydrate (especially refined carbohydrates) diets:

- Diets such as the Atkins diet where carbohydrate is restricted to just 20 grams daily for around 2–4 weeks followed by an expansion to 40 g for a few more weeks depending on progress. This then goes on to 60 g a day, again, depending on progress, but you may need to restrict your diet for several months.

- Much less restricted is a diet which takes into account the glycaemic index (GI) of various foods. The GI is a measure of how fast a particular carbohydrate is absorbed. Foods with a low GI help to keep insulin levels consistent and normal.

- A variant of the low GI diet is the 'low glycaemic load diet'. In this diet foods are assessed slightly differently. The rating is obtained by multiplying the GI index by the available carbohydrate of a specific food. The available carbohydrate does not include non-digestible components such as fibre. Hence, the GI score is divided by 100 and multiplied by the available carbohydrate expressed in grams. I did not become aware of this concept until after I retired, so I was not able to 'road test' it on people who might have benefited from it. The nutritionist, Patrick Holford, has written a very detailed approach called *The Low GL Bible*.

- High-protein/low-fat/low-carbohydrate diets, such as *Protein Power* (1996) and *The Dukan Diet* (2000). Any of these diets will, of course, be considerably more restrictive than the high-protein/high-fat diet. It seems to me that the main advantage of a high-protein/low-fat diet is that it shouldn't attract any disapproval from the cholesterol lobby, and therefore will sell more copies. I would recommend a high-protein diet only to someone who cannot overcome decades of brainwashing on the dangers of fat. Personally I do not see any advantage to diets containing only high protein with little fat and it is dangerous to eat like this for more than seven days at a time.

I will therefore restrict my further comments to the Atkins diet and the low GI diet.

The Atkins diet: general considerations

As the Atkins diet is both the most famous and arguably the most well-constructed low-carbohydrate diet, I would like to discuss the broad outlines, although I would recommend patients to purchase a copy of the original work if they elect to follow it.

Dr Robert Atkins was a cardiologist and a full-time practising physician with lots of practical experience of managing problems of heart disease and obesity. This diet was always bound to upset a lot of physicians devoted to the low-fat/low-calorie concept despite the evidence that such diets are useless in the long term. Doctors addicted to the cholesterol theory were appalled at the thought of their patients eating lots of fat which they had been telling them for many years was highly dangerous. I can visualise countless physicians in the western world clasping their hands in front of them, looking over their glasses, and in the most sombre tones they could muster saying: 'But you must realise that this diet is extremely dangerous even if you have lost two stone in eight weeks, feel enormously better and your blood test results are the best they have ever been.' I imagine that many patients would have lost the confidence to continue at this point, devastated that the only diet that had ever helped them was being forbidden. From vast clinical experience, as a general rule, I have found that if a person ever finds a approach that makes them feels significantly better they should stay with it.

The 'dangers' of this diet are, in my view, totally unfounded. Atkins was basically telling his readers to return to the type of diet that was eaten by our ancestors before grains became a major part of daily life.

Summary of the Atkins diet

The Atkins diet was originally published in the 1970s and has become progressively better in subsequent editions. With more experience, Dr Atkins was able to address most of the situations that can cause problems. Basically, the diet comprises four phases. It starts relatively strictly and then expands as your weight decreases. The first phase lasts around two weeks. In this phase the person is restricted to:

- all meats
- all fish
- most shellfish
- eggs
- cream (2-3 tablespoons a day)
- hard cheeses (though limited to some extent)
- vegetable oils (preferably cold pressed)
- butter
- salad vegetables up to 8 oz a day
- other low carbohydrate vegetables up to 7 oz
- decaffeinated tea or coffee.

If you go onto the induction phase you may have some adverse symptoms for the first four or five days which may be due to withdrawal from food sensitivity or to ketosis. If any possible food sensitivities have already been sorted out the symptoms will probably be mild and due to ketosis.

Ketosis

Ketosis is the condition that usually occurs after two to three days on the induction phase of the Atkins diet, and is caused by the low levels of carbohydrates that are being consumed. Ketones are excreted in the urine and often in the breath. These chemicals are a direct by-product of breaking down fat in your adipose tissue. Some people complain of bad breath but in fact this mechanism results in a sweet odour on the breath. This is an extremely normal and non-toxic phenomenon. In truth it is great in that it indicates you are burning fat big time. This process is called 'lipolysis' (burning up fat). The result is ketosis. Ketosis is sometimes confused with 'ketoacidosis', which is, in fact, a completely different process. Ketoacidosis is a complication of type I diabetes, with insulin deficiency leading to out of control blood sugar levels.

Ketosis can be measured using strips that are dipped into the urine and change colour according to the level of substance that is being measured, in this case ketones. These are called 'Ketostix' in the UK and 'Lipolytic Testing Strips' in the US. These sticks turn to pink initially and then progressively darker to purple as the person goes further into ketosis. It is not essential to use these sticks, which can be easily obtained from any pharmacist, but it does add to the interest. After five days the person should be showing obvious weight loss and the Ketostix will be showing purple. If this isn't happening it can be because of one of two reasons. Firstly, you may be inadvertently eating more carbohydrates than you realise and will need to check labels carefully or use more accurate scales. Secondly, it may mean that this approach is not a suitable strategy for you in particular.

I found men usually lose 10-12 lb (4.5–5.5 kg) in the first two weeks. For some reason, women usually lose only 5–7 lb (2.25–3 kg). I know this is very unfair, but I am not sure what the reason is. If you are very overweight the weight loss can be very much higher.

The initial induction phase is then followed by:

- the on-going weight loss phase
- the pre-maintenance phase
- the life-time maintenance phase.

In these phases, carbohydrate consumption slowly increases as pancreatic function improves. As I said earlier, if you wish to go on this diet please buy the book for full instructions.

How an 'Atkins-type' diet may not work because of food sensitivities: Eileen B

Eileen B, aged 40, was 30 lb (13.5 kg) overweight, and had headaches and fatigue. She originally saw me in 1996 and went on my elimination diet, noticing distinct withdrawal symptoms of headache and fatigue starting from day one. The symptoms continued up to day five. By day seven she had lost 7 lb (3 kg) weight and felt wonderful. She then reintroduced 50 foods back into her diet, reacting to six of them. By the end of the diet she had lost all of the 30 lb (13.5 kg) excess weight. I desensitised her to the six offending foods, enabling her to continue eating them. For the next year her weight remained stable at an ideal level and there was no recurrence of symptoms.

After about a year some of her symptoms started to come back and her weight increased. I suggested she return to the clinic and have her neutralising levels re-tested, which she did. Within a few days of taking the new vaccine her symptoms receded and her weight returned to her ideal. Obviously her neutralising level for a couple of foods had changed over time, which can happen, as explained in detail in chapter 6.

After a further year the same thing happened, and if she had rung me I would have suggested she should have her neutralising levels checked again or avoid the foods she had previously identified as problems. Instead, she was persuaded by a friend to try the Atkins diet. This she did, but after two weeks she had lost only 2 lb (as opposed to losing 7 lb (3 kg) in just one week on the elimination diet). She also had headaches and fatigue.

At this stage she came to see me again. Looking through her notes I noticed that on the elimination diet she had reacted to milk and eggs as well as four other foods.I asked her if she had eaten eggs or milk products on the Atkins induction phase. She replied she had. She had forgotten that she had been sensitive to these foods as she had been successfully taking the neutralising vaccines, which enabled her to eat them without any adverse effect. In fact the neutralisation had been so successful she had completely forgotten which foods were identified originally.

Eileen, therefore, never really needed to embark on a low-carbohydrate diet as managing her food sensitivities had sorted out the whole problem.

'Why did I do so well initially on a low-carb diet, then it all went pear-shaped?'

I have heard this wailed at me on so many occasions. A person may do well on the first phase of the Atkins diet because s/he is not sensitive to any of the foods permitted. However, on a later phase, a food to which s/he is sensitive may be re-introduced without the person noticing a problem on the initial re-introduction. This could be because s/he is not expecting or looking out for a food reaction. Alternatively, the person may have developed a tolerance to a food not eaten for some weeks during the first phase, so when the food is re-introduced no immediate reaction occurs, but the tolerance is lost when the food is once again eaten on a regular basis (see chapter 4 for more details).

The glycaemic index approach

The glycaemic index approach should be used as a useful tool for weight maintenance. Carbohydrates can be eaten, but are best eaten only in their natural unrefined state.

The concept of a glycaemic index (GI) was originally conceived by Dr Gerald Reaven to reinforce the concept that the high speed of absorption of refined carbohydrates was extremely important. Other researchers, at Oxford University, developed the scores listed below by measuring blood sugar levels two hours after consuming specific foods. At first they evaluated the reaction to a solution of glucose alone to provide a standard with which to compare other foods. Glucose was allocated the number 100. Only maltose (in beer) had a higher reading, of 110; this was probably because all alcoholic drinks have very high absorbability. All other foods absorb more slowly; the slower the response, the lower the number. Obviously, from what I have explained earlier, it is healthier to eat the ones with the lower numbers. Generally speaking, the foods that have a glycaemic index under 50 are the best to choose. One fact that this approach emphasises is that the preparation of individual foods has a great influence on how fast the carbohydrate enters the bloodstream. For example, raw carrots have a GI of 30 whereas cooked (boiled) carrots have a GI of 85. More examples are:

Potatoes	- unpeeled and boiled	65
	- peeled and boiled	70
	- instant mashed potato mix	90
	- potato crisps	90
	- chips	95
	- sauté potatoes	95
Rice		
	- wild	35
	- brown (wholegrain)	50

- basmati	50
- long grain rice	60
- pudding rice	70
- puffed rice	85
- rice pudding	85
- ground rice	95

Cereal grains

- 100% wholemeal bread	40
- wholegrain pasta (al dente)	50
- bran bread	50
- white spaghetti	55
- mixed flour bread	65
- refined cereals with sugar	70
- ravioli	70
- white bread baguette	70
- corn flakes	85
- pop corn	85
- burger bun	85

Sugars

- glucose	100
- fructose	20
- table sugar (sucrose)	70
- high fructose corn sugar	55
- maltose (in beer)	110

Values of other items that you might find interesting are:

Fruit and vegetables

- green leafy vegetables	<15
- tomatoes	<15
- aubergine	<15
- courgettes	<15
- garlic	<15
- onions	<15

- fresh apricots	15
- soya / peanuts	15
- green beans	15
- many fresh fruits	30
- figs / dried apricots	35
- kidney beans	40
- fresh peas	40
- banana	60
- melon	60
- turnips	65
- granulated / caster sugar (sucrose)	70
- water melon	75
- cooked broad beans	80
Other items	
- milk products	30
- honey	85
- modified starch	95

One of the drawbacks to the glycaemic index is that food combinations such as ice cream have a GI of only 40. This is because a proportion of it is fat which has no GI at all, the rest is of course sugar with a high GI. It is, however, misleading for people to consider ice cream as a healthy option.

Reasons to avoid high-fructose corn syrup (HFCS55)

The really serious problem with the glycaemic index is fructose (mostly found in fruits), which has a GI of only 20, while sucrose scores 70 and glucose (mostly found in manufactured products such as chocolate) is 100. It is perfectly true that fructose does not have any substantial role in raising blood sugar levels. This fact was seized upon by several soft drink manufacturers so they produced a 'sugar' called high-fructose corn syrup (glucose) which was composed of 55% fructose and 45% glucose. This became known as HFCS55. Doing this gave a product with a GI of approximately 55, which appears much better than the 100 of the original glucose, particularly as it tastes the same as pure glucose.

In 1978, HFCS55 was marketed to the public as an excellent alternative to conventional sugar. You might think this sounds like a good idea, but in fact it is much worse as the body is a complicated machine and things are not quite so straightforward as they seem at first.

The glucose component passes straight into the bloodstream (hence high GI) and is taken up by the tissues for immediate energy usage. Only 35% of the ingested glucose goes into the liver. All of the fructose, however, goes straight into the liver (hence much lower GI). Why is this a problem, you might ask? Firstly, as the fructose is completely metabolised by the liver it imposes a heavy burden on that organ. Secondly, the liver rapidly converts the fructose to the type of fat called triglycerides. As we have seen (see page 172), triglycerides are a well-known risk factor for coronary artery disease, but from a weight management point of view they are particularly harmful as they are immediately sent straight to the fatty tissues for storage. This is known to the medical profession as 'fructose induced lipogenesis'.

Fructose thus stimulates the liver to produce triglycerides, and at the same time the glucose leads to high insulin levels which then further stimulate the liver to produce even higher triglyceride levels. It is therefore a double whammy. Triglyceride levels are ever more being linked to obesity and coronary artery disease. This is the main reason why triglyceride levels drop like a stone on low-carbohydrate diets such as the Atkins diet.

Table sugar is labelled as sucrose, but sucrose is, in fact, a combination of both glucose and fructose that are chemically bound together. Digestion breaks the bond and the component parts then behave as explained above.

Recent work at the University of California has confirmed that fructose is more readily converted into fat, in the liver, than glucose. This can lead to liver disease, type II diabetes and eventually heart disease in some people. New fat cells gather around the heart and digestive organs. In California they have found that feeding patients neat glucose instead of fructose produced far fewer problems, although glucose is a long way from being a health food.

Fructose is, of course, present in fruits so the obvious question is whether it is dangerous to eat lots of fruit. In my view eating fruit is not a big problem unless you already have a much damaged liver and pancreas. Apart from anything else, the fruit contains a lot of fibre and pectin which will delay the absorption of the fructose. However, concentrated fruit juices are a different matter. A large glass of fresh orange juice may contain the equivalent of six whole oranges which would be almost impossible to eat in one sitting. Bear in mind that our ancestors only ate fruits in season, which would only have been a few months a year.

More seriously, this high-fructose corn syrup is present in a whole range of cereals and soft drinks. Most commonly it is described as glucose/fructose syrup or HFCS or HFCS55. It has many advantages to food manufacturers as it is cheap, and boosts shelf life by keeping food moist. In the USA some manufacturers are removing HFCS55 from their products and returning to straight sugar. This is due to adverse publicity related to, what in the USA, has been dubbed the 'devil's candy'.

There are a number of foods that contain this product in the UK, though, hopefully, the situation may soon change.

Why beer deserves a section of its own

The sugar in beer is derived from malt and is called maltose. It has the highest glycaemic index of any food substance, with a GI of 110. Beer is full of this malt sugar, which is exceptionally fattening. The fact that beer contains alcohol is the main reason for its unusually rapid absorption. All alcoholic drinks absorb into the bloodstream very quickly, but wines and spirits don't have anything in them that is so highly fattening. Before 1880 the only people who became significantly obese were usually heavy beer drinkers. Henry VIII is well known for being enormously over-weight in his later life and he allegedly drank around 14 pints of beer a day. Many people who weigh over 30 stone (190 kg) often drink large quantities of beer. Whoever coined the term 'a beer belly' was spot on.

Anyone who is serious about losing weight, and keeping to their ideal weight, should not even think about drinking beer.

Are high-fat/low-carbohydrate diets safe?

When high-fat/low-carbohydrate diets became popular, many physicians were uncomfortable about their patients eating large quantities of protein and fat. Clinical trials were obviously need-ed and fairly soon we had them. In 2002 the University of Con-necticut initiated a study[37] of very-low-carbohydrate/high-fat diets on normal-weight men with normal cholesterol levels. The diet contained only 8% of calories from carbohydrate and 61% from fat. With such a high fat content many cardiologists would have said that the cholesterol levels would have surely rocketed. In fact the opposite occurred. Overall cholesterol levels fell by 29% and the high-density lipoproteins (the so-called 'good' cho-lesterol) went up by 11%. The triglyceride levels, which are the most significant factor in heart disease, reduced by a magnificent 33%, and insulin fell by 34%. These results demonstrated that not only are low carbohydrate diets free from danger, but they are in fact much safer, heart wise, than normal eating.

This study had, however, covered a period of only six weeks, so doctors at Duke University conducted a similar study[38] covering a period of six months. In this study carbohydrates were restricted to only 25 g a day, similar to the induction phase of the Atkins diet (20g). The participants were allowed to eat unlimited amounts of meat, fish, eggs, cheese, butter and other fats. On average they lost 21 lb (9.5 kg) and their cholesterol fell by 6%. There was also a 40% drop in the level of triglycerides, and HDL (good cholesterol) increased by 7%. This Duke University study is typical of many other studies, and not one of them has shown any increase in cholesterol or triglycerides or any lowering of HDL.

'So, Dr Mansfield, how do you see the role of low-carbohydrate diets in managing my weight?'

First of all, as I have said elsewhere in this book, I don't consider that most people need to become involved in low-carbohydrate dieting at all. What I have emphasised throughout this book is that I am not just interested in temporary weight loss, for example for a special occasion. I am interested in permanent weight loss, so that the problem is not an ongoing part of your life, and you can get on with enjoying living. I have achieved this already with countless people.

I know that the Atkins diet has helped millions of people, when other dietary regimes have proved useless. One study at least has demonstrated some disappointing aspects of the long-term effects of the Atkins approach. This study, 'A randomised trial of a low carbohydrate diet for obesity,' was published in the *New England Journal of Medicine*.[39] The conclusion was that this particular diet (Atkins) produced greater weight loss than the conventional low-calorie diet for the first six months, but after one year, although the weight loss was slightly better than with the conventional diet, it was only marginally so.

This was a big let-down to a method which started so promisingly, in my view. The people studied probably had food sensitivities which they didn't recognise when they reintroduced certain foods after many months of avoidance. They probably didn't notice a reaction initially, because the longer you remove a food from your diet the less obvious is the effect. Also, of course, they weren't looking out for reactions.

For this reason I feel strongly that no-one should embark on a low-carbohydrate diet without first having completed my elimination diet to identify any possible food sensitivities.

A small proportion of people with major weight problems manage to lose a great deal of weight on the elimination diet and/or the yeast syndrome diet, but still have further weight to lose. After many years of consuming large amounts of refined carbohydrates these people often end up with damage to their pancreases. In this situation, it is wise for them to give their pancreas a few months' 'holiday' with one of the low-carbohydrate regimes. This could either be the Atkins diet or the low-glycaemic index diet.

'What if I have a poor response to a low-carbohydrate diet?'

There are a few people who give every indication that they have problems with metabolising fats. If you are one of these people you may be deficient in the amino acid called carnitine which is essential for transporting fatty acids into the mitochondria (the cells' energy producers). This is especially likely if you eat little or no meat, particularly red meat, as meat is the only significant source of this amino acid. Carnitine exists in several forms and supplements are widely available. Another nutrient that may be useful is 'co enzyme Q10'. This is another substance that is important in helping the body to burn energy.

It is also possible that if you have problems burning fat you may respond to a diet low in both carbohydrates and fats – that is, an all-protein diet, such as the Dukan diet. Such a diet should be followed for no more than seven days at a time.

People who seem unable to burn fat are thankfully rare and can be a major challenge to the medical profession. I do not think that science has uncovered all of the answers to this problem as yet.

The low-fat/high-carbohydrate catastrophe

The American clinical obesity level throughout the 1960s and '70s was fairly stable at around 13% of the population. After 1978 this level escalated rapidly. The figure increased to 21% in the '80s and '90s, but by 2005 it was 33%. I regard the 20% increase in obesity levels since 1978 as the 'American Mega Epidemic'.

Figures 10.2, 10.3 and 10.4 come from American governmental statistics. Figure 10.2 shows the increase in weight problems in the US population between 1960 and 2002. Although the percentage of calories that they ate from fat had steadily decreased (see Figures 10.3 and 10.4) the percentage of people that were obese increased markedly.

Figure 10.2: American statistics demonstrating the distinct rise in the rate of obesity after the 1970s (from the Centers for Disease Control and Prevention, National Center for Health Statistics, US, 2005)

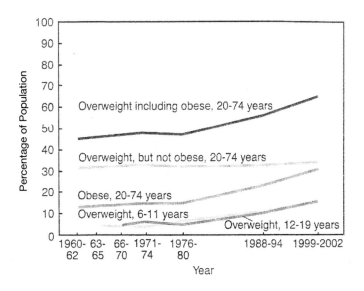

Figure 10.3: The changes in the source of calories as eaten by women aged 20-74 between 1971 and 2000

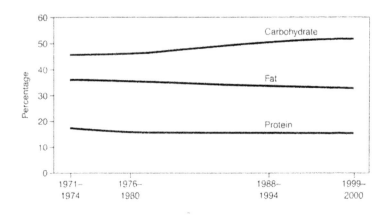

Figure 10.4: The changes in the source of calories as eaten by men aged 20-74 between 1971 and 2000

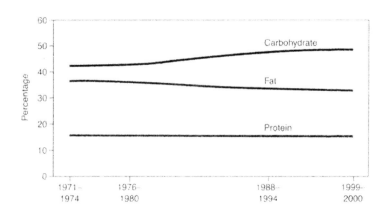

I think there were two main reasons for this great increase in weight in the USA starting at the end of the 1970s. As you can see, fat consumption steadily declined while carbohydrate consumption rapidly increased. Total daily calorie consumption increased on average by 500 calories and 90% of these calories came from carbohydrates. The remaining 10% came from protein and fat.

So what happened? In 1977-1978 there were two events of enormous significance:

- The American Heart Association advised Americans to reduce their fat intake as much as possible, and this they did, spectacularly. They also said, amazingly, that carbohydrates of any type were no problem.
- High-fructose corn syrup (HFCS55) (see page 183) became widely used and represented 90% of the extra carbohydrate consumed. The average consumption of total fat dropped from 113 grams daily in 1977 to 96 grams daily in 1989.

We now have well over 100 million American men, women and children who are clinically obese and this huge surge demonstrated on the graphs above occurred when Americans limited their fat consumption as never before. How much of this increase was due to eating HFC55 and how much to lower amounts of fat in the diet is impossible to estimate. However, many products containing this HFCS55 have now been withdrawn from the market, in both the USA and the UK.

At virtually the same time as these two factors were affecting the Americans a similar weight epidemic was happening 3000 miles across the Atlantic in the UK. In the UK, the effects of the cholesterol theory were in full swing and vast numbers of people changed to low fat diets from the late 1970s onwards. According to the *British Medical Journal*, in just 11 years (1980-1991) the incidence of obesity doubled. The remarkable difference between the UK and USA was that the British people had reduced their total intake of calories by 20%, whereas the Americans had increased their daily intake by 500 calories, exclusively by eating more carbohydrates. Exercise levels also increased in those same

11 years. So, to summarise, in those 11 years, people in the UK exercised more, ate 20% fewer calories and restricted fat consumption as never before, yet obesity rates doubled.

Why am I so convinced that it is following a low-fat diet that has caused so many people to become fatter to the point of obesity? First, there is the amazingly consistent time correlation between these obesity epidemics and the onset of low-fat dieting. Secondly, and just as convincing, is the day-to-day observation of the difference that occurs when people have adequate amounts of fat in their diet, and when they don't. The fact that fat has a major satiating effect can be observed easily.

Anyone who has a breakfast of refined cereals and sugar will have a sharp rise in blood sugar (and hence insulin), which will drop rapidly three to four hours later, and will induce food cravings. Many people, for this reason, carry a carbohydrate snack to rescue them from this mid-morning 'hypo'. After a breakfast of, say,. eggs and bacon alone, there will only be a minimal rise in blood sugar and insulin levels. Consequently, there will be no rapid drop after three to four hours, with the usual food cravings. Instead, there is a transition into normal hunger around lunch time.

Anyone with the low-fat eating habit is likely to spend their life with wildly swinging blood glucose levels, which can dominate their whole being. Considering the vast increase in illness associated with obesity it is surely time for the medical professions in both America and the UK to admit that this advice, while initially given in good faith, has been proved wrong. If the advice is not changed we shall soon see rates of clinical obesity in the USA climbing to over 40%, thus leading to the current generation living shorter lives than their parents.

This chapter began with the story of William Banting, the undertaker with enormous obesity cured by a low-carbohydrate diet in 1862. This was followed by his letter on 'Corpulence' addressed to the public. This approach was used by doctors to help patients towards reasonable control of their weight for over 100 years. In the last 50 years, with notable exceptions, much of the western world has chosen to ignore this relatively successful approach and advise the complete opposite, that is, major fat limitation but limitless amounts of any carbohydrate. Despite the fact that we know all the science behind the successful low carbohydrate approach it has been ignored leading to, perhaps, the greatest self-inflicted medical disaster in history.

Chapter summary

- In 1862, William Banting published the first book to recommend a low-fat diet for successful weight loss.
- For the next 100 years, doctors used such diets.
- During this time, there were quite a lot of overweight people, but nothing like the pandemic that has occurred since the late 1970s.
- Low-fat diets were adopted from the late 1970s as a result of the 'cholesterol theory', which blamed heart disease on saturated fats and were endorsed by the American Heart Association. Since that time, obesity levels in the UK and the USA have trebled.
- Clinical trials evaluating low-carbohydrate diets have all shown that this dietary approach is successful, producing both major weight loss and a reduction in stored body fat without the loss of muscle.
- Dr Mackarness's book *Eat Fat and Grow Slim* advocated low-carbohydrate diets in 1957, but the best-known books on the subject are by Dr Robert Atkins.
- For people who still have weight to lose after the elimination diet and treating the yeast syndrome, I recommend an Atkins-type diet or a low-GI (glycaemic index) diet.
- It has been known for many years that diabetes and heart disease are often associated with major weight problems.

- In the 1970s, 'insulin resistance' was recognised as the cause of type II diabetes by the American Diabetic Association. In insulin resistance, ever higher amounts of insulin are needed to produce the body's normal response to carbohydrates, as a result of over-consuming refined carbohydrates.
- Patients who have survived heart attacks have been found to have high levels of triglycerides and problems dealing with glucose, both of which are associated with insulin resistance. This suggests insulin resistance, caused only by eating too many refined carbohydrates, is a major cause of heart disease.
- Thus weight gain, diabetes and heart disease have nothing to do with eating fat. Diabetes is caused by the over-consumption of refined sugar, and coronary artery disease by all refined carbohydrates plus cigarette smoking.

Chapter 11

The nutritional consequences of eating refined carbohydrates

In the last 40 years research in nutritional medicine has come on in leaps and bounds. This has been, helped, in no small part, by our ability now to measure levels of trace minerals, vitamins, essential fatty acids, amino acids and other important nutrients. They can be measured in the blood, urine and even sweat.

The first nutritional laboratory to open its doors in the UK was the Biolab Medical Unit, in London in 1982. Although I was heavily involved in allergy my knowledge of nutritional medicine, like most doctors, was virtually nil until Biolab opened. (During my student days at Guy's Hospital we had only four or five lectures on nutritional matters during the whole five years of training. I do remember they were not particularly useful or memorable.)

With this basis, nutritional medicine has given us an understanding of the consequences of eating refined carbohydrates.

Chromium deficiency

Chromium is the most important trace mineral in relation to weight problems, diabetes, and coronary artery disease. This mineral has been recognised as essential to health since 1960, and yes, it is the same metal that can end up on your car. It acts primarily to regulate the action of insulin which you will know from the last chapter is the key to everything concerning weight, diabetes and to a significant extent, coronary artery disease.

In the past, various researchers into nutrition had noted that as people aged in the UK and USA they appeared to have progressively diminished levels of chromium (in blood and sweat samples). Biolab verified this observation[40] in 1997 by referring to its vast database of 40,800 patients who had attended its clinic between 1985 and 1996. This laboratory keeps, anonymously, all of its patient data. Its test results showed a reduction of 46% in chromium levels between birth and the age of 75. Interestingly, in the USA the findings are similar. This reduction is not found in the Far East, presumably because they have nothing like the amount of refined carbohydrates that we do in the UK and USA.

Natural sugars and grains do contain a great deal of chromium which aids the metabolism of these foods. However, almost all of the chromium is lost during the refining process of both sugar and flour. As we have already seen, there has been a vast increase in the consumption of sugar in British and American diets, while the consumption of fat has not increased at all over the past 100 years. Refined-sugar (sucrose) intake has increased by 1000%. Sucrose is composed of glucose and fructose and does nothing other than supply calories. It makes no contribution to levels of essential nutrients.

The Miami Heart Institute reviewed all published papers[41] on the role of chromium depletion in diabetes and arterial sclerosis (hardening of the arteries). It concluded that adequate levels of chromium were vital to preventing these conditions.

The diagram (Figure 10.1) in the last chapter showing the consequences of eating refined carbohydrates can now be extended as follows:

Figure 11.1: Diagram showing how chromium deficiency is part of the pathway from eating refined carbohydrates to eventually getting coronary artery disease

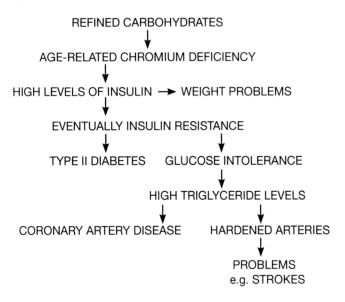

These processes have the following consequences:
- 40% of people, in addition to diabetics, over the age of 40 have abnormal glucose tolerance tests. 50% of these people have been shown to improve with chromium supplementation. This means they are better able to handle glucose and far less likely to develop diabetes at a later date.[42]
- In several studies people who died of coronary thrombosis were found to have very low chromium in their aortas (largest blood vessel in the body that leads from the heart). Accident victims usually had normal chromium levels in their aortas.[43]
- Feeding animals chromium-deficient diets caused diabetes, and the diabetes was cured by the reintroduction of chromium.

I have personally found that giving chromium picolinate at a dose of 200 μg twice a day, combined with a low refined-carbohydrate diet, to diabetics who had not yet become insulin dependent led to a resolution of their type II diabetes.

I was particularly pleased when I treated a friend of mine who had just been told by the local hospital that he had diabetes at the age of 55. He was told that they would try the oral diabetic drugs for a couple of months, but he would soon need to go onto insulin. I sent him to the Biolab laboratory and found his sweat and red blood cell levels of chromium were both low. I gave him chromium picolinate. His blood levels of sugar started to decrease so he reduced his oral diabetic drugs from three daily to two daily and then one daily. He was monitoring his blood sugar levels daily and I told him at which point to reduce his medication. Roughly, he was able to decrease the dosage by one a week until they were no longer necessary as his blood sugar continued to be in the normal range.

He went back to the diabetic clinic at the hospital for assessment after two months. They told him he had had a fantastic response to the drugs. He told them he wasn't taking them any more, just chromium. We remained friends for many years after, in which time he continued to take the chromium and the diabetes never returned. I sent the hospital a nice letter, and a copy of several studies on chromium but they were not interested. A case of cognitive dissonance (the inability to hold two incompatible beliefs simultaneously).

There have been countless studies confirming the benefits of chromium in the treatment of diabetes. If you are interested try looking up Dr R A Anderson and chromium on the internet.

B vitamin deficiencies and homocysteine

Fairly soon after the refining of grains began in the mid-1800s, there were major outbreaks of conditions caused by vitamin B deficiencies. The removal of vitamin B_1 (thiamine) in the refining process led to beri beri. The loss of vitamin B_3 (niacin) led to pellagra. Eventually these problems were mostly resolved by adding these specific vitamins to flour and rice. But what of the other B vitamins – especially B_6 and B_9 – that are also removed along with the husk and the fibre?

It would be nearly a century before it was discovered how vital a role the B vitamins play in keeping the heart healthy. Dr Kilmer McCully's book *The Homocysteine Revolution* published in 1997 proved to be a major breakthrough in the understanding of heart disease and stroke. In 1968, while working as a researcher at Harvard University, Dr McCully came across the cases of two young children, both of whom had died from massive strokes. This is, of course, virtually unheard of at a very young age. At post-mortem they both appeared to have exceptionally advanced hardening and narrowing of their arteries. Both children had a very rare genetic disease called homocysteineuria. This disease is so named because patients' urine contains a very high level of an amino acid called homocysteine. They have this condition because they lack an enzyme (called cystathione synthase) which has to be present to convert homocysteine (which is toxic) to the non-toxic cystathione. Homocysteine is a normal metabolic by-product of eating protein that the body can deal with efficiently when the correct enzymes are present. What McCully wondered was whether this rare and fatal condition of children could give a major insight into the cause of coronary artery disease and stroke in adults.

It had already been discovered that these children could be helped, to some extent, by giving them high doses of vitamin B_6. This helps reduce the amount of homocysteine in the urine. He identified that B_{12} and folic acid (B_9) were also crucial.

To illustrate the significance of homocysteine in general health I would like briefly to describe a trial carried out in Norway in 1992. This study[44] involved 4766 people initially aged 65–67 over a period of five years. Each person had their homocysteine level measured at the beginning. Over the next five years, 162 of the men and 97 of the women died. When the statistics of the study were analysed it was found that a reduction of just five units (see later explanation) in their homocysteine score had the effect of reducing the risk of death by the following:

- 49% from all causes
- 50% from heart disease
- 26% from cancer
- 104% from any cause of death other than heart disease or cancer.

Needless to say, this subject has exploded far outside the confines of coronary heart disease and strokes. There are now thousands of clinical studies on homocysteine related to cancer, dementias, depression, fatigue and multitudes of other conditions.

'Methylation' and 'anti-oxidation and detoxification' are two major biochemical processes by which your body, if working well and in balance, largely controls how slowly/rapidly you age and how soon you may suffer chronic disease. Your homocysteine level indicates how well these processes are working and explains why high homocysteine levels can indicate a predisposition to a very wide range of illnesses.

Most people can now jump to the section 'Should I get my homocysteine level measured?' (see page 202). However, if you are the sort of person who wants to know all of the details, then I am about to outline the biochemistry of this subject.

Metabolising the amino acid methionine

Amino acids are the building blocks of all protein. Meat, fish, cheese and other milk products are very rich in the amino acid 'methionine', and it is therefore usually eaten daily.

In the normal course of events, methionine is converted into another amino acid called homocysteine. This is the starting point for the two biochemical processes already mentioned:

'methylation' and 'anti-oxidation and detoxification'. Between them, these two processes control a vast amount of the biochemistry that goes on in our bodies every second of the day.

Methylation

In the methylation process, 'methyl groups', which consist of one carbon atom and three hydrogen atoms, are added to, or subtracted from, other molecules. This enables the body to make all sorts of vital substances, such as hormones.

Two enzymes are essential for this process. One is called 'methyltransferase' and the other has such a long name that it is known by its initials, MTHFR. The first enzyme needs folic acid (vitamin B_9), vitamin B_{12}, vitamin B_2 and zinc to work properly. If these are in short supply methylation does not work well. The other enzyme needs vitamin B_{12} and trimethyl glycine (known as a methyl donor). This pathway eventually produces a substance (known as SAMe) which organises all the methylation processes in our bodies.

Anti-oxidation and detoxification

The anti-oxidation and detoxification process begins with sulphur being added to homocysteine via an enzyme called cystathione beta synthase, which needs adequate amounts of vitamins B_6, B_2, and zinc. Another enzyme, called 'cystathione lysase', which also needs vitamins B_6, B_2 and zinc, completes the transition to glutathione (which is another essential amino acid). Glutathione is the key to the body's anti-ageing and chemical detoxification processes.

If you are deficient in any of the nutrients concerned, these vital pathways function poorly and as a consequence your level of homocysteine rises, indicating that there is trouble afoot.

'Should I get my homocysteine level measured?'

Basically the answer is 'yes', as it is one of the most useful tests in the whole of preventive medicine. However, currently it is only available on the NHS to patients who have warning signs of coronary artery disease – for example, patients who already suffer from angina, or who have been admitted to hospital. Although routinely done in hospitals for patients who already have some cardiac problems, it is rarely done as a screening procedure. It is possible you may succeed in convincing your own GP to send you for a blood test at the local hospital, particularly if you are over 50. If you feel you can afford to have the test done privately there are a number of laboratories offering this service.

The units that homocysteine are measured in are millimoles (mmol/l). A low level that is ideal would be around 6 mmol/l; an average would be around 10-11 mmol/l; over 15 mmol/l would be high; if you are over 20 mmol/l, it is serious. The interpretation of these levels varies somewhat from one specialist to another.

Various companies making nutritional supplements manufacture the ideal combination of vitamins B_6 and B_{12}, folic acid (B_9), zinc and trimethylglycine (TMG) specifically designed to lower homocysteine. The formulation by each company is more or less the same. I have listed a few in appendix II. The usual dosage is as follows:

- Blood level 6-9 mmol/l (low risk) – 1 cap twice daily
- Blood level 9-15 mmol/l (moderate risk) – 2 caps twice daily
- Blood level above 15 mmol/l (high risk) – 3 caps twice daily

If you are unable to get your homocysteine level measured it is a good preventative measure to take one capsule twice daily. B vitamins are important for many other bodily functions and are completely non-toxic.

Proof that lowering homocysteine helps prevent heart disease and strokes

The largest study ever completed on the relationship between homocysteine levels and heart disease and strokes was performed by one of Britain's leading cardiologists, Dr David Wald, at Southampton University's Department of Cardiology. This was reported in the *British Medical Journal*[45] in 2002 and was an analysis of 92 studies that measured homocysteine levels in over 20,000 people. Some people carry a gene that predisposes them to have greater problems with homocysteine than the average population. For every increase of 5 mmol/l of homocysteine, the risk of heart disease went up by 42% for those people with the predisposing gene, and 32% for those without it.

When it came to cerebral vascular disease (strokes) the risk went up by a massive 65% in those with the genetic mutation, and by 59% in those without, again with each increase of 5 mmol/l. This demonstrates that reducing the level of homocysteine in the blood is by far the most effective way of preventing strokes.

Perhaps an even better example of how beneficial it is to keep homocysteine levels low was a study by Kilmer McCully and FM Ellis,[46] published in 1995. They reported that just taking the recommended daily dose of vitamin B_6 and folic acid led to a 73% reduction in the risk of angina and coronary thrombosis with an average increase in lifespan of eight years.

These are two of many studies that confirm that the relationship between homocysteine and coronary artery disease is not just an association, but is quite definitely one of cause and effect. There are, actually, over 5000 papers exploring the involvement of homocysteine in a wide range of medical conditions. I have a feeling that cardiology and other research departments are sick to death of evaluating the cholesterol theory and are finding this field much more exciting as it is more valuable.

Figure 11.2: How stripping B vitamins from white flour can contribute to coronary artery disease and strokes. (NB Vitamin B_{12} is NOT found in grain. You must eat plenty of meat – especially offal – and dairy products to get enough of it.)

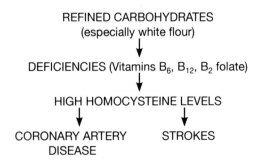

REFINED CARBOHYDRATES
(especially white flour)
↓
DEFICIENCIES (Vitamins B_6, B_{12}, B_2 folate)
↓
HIGH HOMOCYSTEINE LEVELS
↓   ↓
CORONARY ARTERY   STROKES
DISEASE

Chapter summary

- There have been major increases in our ability to understand nutritional medicine in the last 30 years, thanks largely to our being able to measure levels of vitamins, minerals, amino acids and essential fatty acids in blood, urine and sweat. Correcting these levels has played a huge part in understanding the fundamental causes of a great deal of human illness.
- Chromium deficiency plays a major role in diabetes and coronary artery disease as well as weight problems.
- Nearly all of the chromium in raw cane sugar is lost in the refining process.
- We now know that refining food and removing essential nutrients can have significant long-term health consequences.
- The homocysteine theory has been developed over the past 30 to 40 years: it blames overly high levels of the amino acid homocysteine for heart disease and strokes. Homocysteine is derived from protein and is one step on the pathway of proteins being digested, used and excreted by the body.

- Certain B vitamins are essential for homocysteine to be processed by the body; during processing and refining, the B vitamin content is considerably reduced in many foods.
- Clinical studies have now shown that giving people B vitamins not only corrects homocysteine levels, but can also increase life expectancy by seven to eight years.
- A high level of homocysteine is now established as a cause of coronary artery disease as well as strokes, and this role is now discussed in major medical textbooks.
- The cholesterol theory has only ever been established as an association, not a cause.

Chapter 12

Weight gain, diabetes and coronary artery disease are a man-made disaster

In the past, when the great epidemics, like bubonic plague, small-pox, tuberculosis, leprosy and cholera, hit the human race with devastating effects, people had very little hope of dealing with them. The causes of all these diseases were originally not at all understood. The only thing that became fairly apparent was that they were contagious and the avoidance of contact was about the only strategy that helped. Eventually, the causes – various infective organisms – became known and the development of vaccinations and antibiotics has made it possible almost to eradicate these conditions in most parts of the world.

The seeds of the modern epidemics of obesity, diabetes and coronary artery disease were first sown in the period 1850–70. Refined sugar, refined flour and refined rice do not occur at all in nature, and until man made the decision to refine these products, they were never eaten. The refining process strips them of almost all of their nutritional content, leaving just empty calories. During this period there was no sign of diabetes or coronary artery disease and obesity was rare.

For thousands of years whole grains and brown rice had been consumed. Unrefined sugar had also been available for around 200 years, but it was very expensive and only eaten in small quantities, mostly by the very rich. Refined sugar, refined flour and white rice all had two things in common. One was that they all were digested and absorbed into the bloodstream with unprecedented speed. There had previously been no time in history when the human pancreas had been forced to deal with such a massive strain on its function. The other was that they all had greatly reduced chromium content. Refining sugar leads to a 98% reduction in this essential trace mineral, which is vital for the proper metabolism of sugar and the regulation of insulin. This is crucial in weight problems, diabetes and coronary artery disease.

Refining whole grains leads to an extensive loss of most of the B vitamins; an early consequence of this, as described in previous chapters, was the appearance of the disease pellagra. This was eventually traced to a lack of vitamin B_3 (niacin). Later, deficiencies in vitamin B_1 (thiamine) led to the disease beri beri as a consequence of refining brown rice. Very much later, in 1969, Dr Kilmer McCully made the discovery that deficiencies in B_6, folic acid (B_9), and vitamin B_{12} (which is found in meat, sea food and dairy products) were the cause of high levels of homocysteine, a major factor in the development of coronary artery disease (see chapter 11).

Cigarette smoking increased through the 1900s. We therefore had the three major culprits – insulin resistance, the homocysteine problem and cigarette smoking – all rising at the same time. I will describe the effects of cigarette smoking in relation to coronary artery disease later in this chapter. Of course, cigarettes are an entirely man-made concoction.

Technical innovation

In modern times, Europe and the USA have been two of the greatest technical innovators in the world, and this has been largely responsible for their commercial successes. Computers, the internet, mobile phones, television and countless other advances have made our lives much easier and more interesting.

As food is an important part of our lives it is not surprising that there would be a desire to innovate in this area. Breakfast cereals, biscuits, cakes, ice cream, pizzas and the like did not exist in meaningful quantities prior to 1850 and many did not make an appearance before the 1950s. All are based on refined carbohydrates.

Major changes in what we eat are not, in my opinion, a good idea and are fraught with danger. Human beings, like all animals, have always initially reacted adversely to major changes in their diet. When whole grains were first introduced 10,000 years ago there was a marked decrease in life expectancy and a reduction in average height of over five inches. Eventually, over a period of thousands of years human beings partially adapted to whole grains such as wheat, corn (maize), oats, rye and rice. Nevertheless, even nowadays these foods are amongst the most common that people are sensitive to. This is attributable as well to the fact that they are also the most commonly eaten.

Our species has certainly not adapted to white sugar, white flour and white rice, which have been eaten only for, at most, 160 years.

We are genetically programmed to eat meat, fish, vegetables, fruit and nuts. The more we stick to these natural foods, the better our health. As long as you don't have a specific sensitivity to any of the grains, milk or eggs you should be able to eat them too, provided the grains are in their natural unrefined form.

Modern cereal breakfasts versus the 'traditional' breakfast

Nothing illustrates the changes in the western diet more vividly than the arrival of modern cereal breakfasts in the 1960s. Before these arrived there was no such thing as convenience food. In the last 50 to 60 years these products have transformed cheap commodities, such as grains, into hugely profitable brands.

Many of these foods are highly processed. Take, for example the manufacture of corn flakes. Initially the kernel of the corn is removed and then the germ, the oil in which would otherwise go rancid. Next the skin is removed as this allows the flavours – sugar, salt and malt – to penetrate the corn flake. What is left is rolled, cooked and dried down. Finally, the finished product is toasted and, critically, sugar is added, as taste-wise corn flakes are quite unappetising, especially to children.

A kilo of corn (maize) cost 15 p in 2010 and at the same time a kilo of corn flakes, when bought on the high street, cost around £3. Despite the fact that this does not include the cost of the sugar, this vast profit margin allows for hugely expensive advertising campaigns. These campaigns are mostly on television to reach the widest audience. Other objects of added 'value' include cartoon characters on the packets and plastic toys for children. In other words, 'a fun product for the whole family'. They represent what is very quick and easy to prepare, and in various forms are appealing to the whole family.

So what was happening to the traditional English breakfast, usually of eggs in one form or another and bacon? From the beginning, it was losing out as it took much longer to organise and prepare, and many women now had a career as well as a family. The Egg Marketing Board responded in the 1960s with its 'Go to Work on an Egg' advertising campaign, but it didn't stand a chance.

Worst of all was the arrival of the 'cholesterol theory' of heart disease. Eggs contain more cholesterol weight-for-weight than any other food. Bacon was also considered far too high in fat for many people. Eventually, many Americans, in particular, saw eggs and bacon as 'death on a plate'. Recently an American comedian touring England noticed that some Britons were still having the Full English Breakfast when staying at a hotel. He remarked than in America this would now be regarded as a suicide attempt.

Breakfast is a very important meal as it 'sets the scene' diet-wise for the rest of the day. If this meal just contains fat and protein, like egg and bacon, it will cause no rise in blood sugar whatsoever. As a result there will be no rise in insulin levels. If a slice of wholemeal bread is added there will be a slow rise in blood sugar, but not enough to be a problem in any way. The person eating this breakfast will have an appetite that is satisfied till lunch time. However, if refined grains are eaten, like corn-flakes or the many other processed breakfast cereals, plus tea or coffee with sugar, blood sugar levels will rise rapidly. This will then be followed, about two or three hours later, by a rapid fall into hypoglycaemic (very low blood sugar) mode. Mid-morning snacks of confectionary bars, or coffee/tea with sugar, rush to the rescue and the blood sugar again rises. Another couple of hours later the next downturn in blood sugar may be assuaged, by white sandwiches, baguettes, pizza, or the white bun of the hamburger (the hamburger itself is not a problem).

Many people's lives are ruled by these wild fluctuations in their blood sugar, leading to persistently high levels of insulin (hyperinsulinaemia). This may eventually lead to insulin resist-ance, type II diabetes and coronary artery disease.

Problems with the term 'refined carbohydrates'

The term 'refined carbohydrates' is, from a nutritional point of view, rather unfortunate. The adjective 'refined' is generally re-garded as a complimentary term, suggesting improvement and increased sophistication.

Around 1850 the very rich could afford white flour and refined sugar, so the general population aspired to do the same. These items initially were seen as an improvement. Knowl-edge concerning nutritional medicine was very minimal at this time, and the consequences of removing 98% of the chromium from sugar, and most of the B vitamins from flour, might have seemed fairly harmless. In the light of current knowledge the description 'nutritionally stripped carbohydrates' might be more appropriate.

As the medical profession, in general, knows little about nutritional medicine even to this day, it was not appreciated until 1995 that there was a significant difference between unrefined and refined carbohydrates. As such, both refined and unrefined carbohydrates were listed in the nutritional statistics under one heading – 'carbohydrates'. This was a major hindrance in identifying the role of refined carbohydrates in relation to type II diabetes and coronary artery disease.

Low-fat diets

One of the reasons for the high uptake of low-fat diets was that they were very easy to manage, some of the reasons being:
- You can use margarine/spreads instead of butter
- You can easily change from full-fat milk to skimmed milk
- You can choose low-fat yoghurt
- You can replace eggs with breakfast cereal, which also has the advantage of less cooking
- You can cut down on meat consumption.

Most of these strategies will save time and money, and most people also prefer to eat sweet-tasting foods, if permitted to do so. However, the problem with this approach is:
- Margarine is high in 'trans' fats which have been proven to be detrimental to health. Recently, in the UK, the term 'margarine' has disappeared from the products on the supermarket shelves because of all the bad press. It has been replaced by the term 'spread'; these claim not to include hydrogenated oils.
- By eliminating the cream from the milk you are missing out on the fat-soluble vitamins at the same time as getting higher amounts of the milk sugar lactose. This also applies to yoghurt.

- Eggs, in particular, are exquisitely dense in beneficial nutrients.
- Meat is also a very rich source of most important nutrients, especially vitamin B_{12} which is not available in any plant foods.

Margarine itself has proved to be a particularly unhealthy substance. A recent article in the *British Medical Journal*[47] has shown that trans fatty acids cause around 11,000 heart attacks and 7000 avoidable deaths each year in the UK. Similarly in the USA, in a 2006 study,[47] it was found that an intake of five grams of trans fatty acids per day was associated with a 23% increase in coronary artery disease.

Trans fatty acids are popular with the food industry because of their convenience and very low cost. As well as being present in margarine they are also found in many deep-fried foods, bakery products, sweets and snacks, such as biscuits.

One of the heroes of this story is Professor Spender of Copenhagen University who managed to get trans fatty acids totally banned in his native Denmark in 2003. Every foodstuff, including importantly all imports, has since then been free from trans fatty acids, and no one has noticed a change in either taste or price. Switzerland and Austria followed in 2009.

In the USA, the FDA (Food and Drug Administration) has ruled that manufacturers can label their products with the phrase 'Contains No Trans Fats' even if they do contain some, provided there are less than 500 mg per 'serving', whatever a 'serving' might be. However, New York City took matters into its own hands and banned trans fats from being served in any restaurant. The amount of trans fats in cooking oil then fell from 50% to 2%. Seattle and Baltimore followed suit and no major manufacturer can ignore cities of this size. For example, the trans fat content of chicken nuggets and chips from McDonalds and Kentucky Fried Chicken food chains has been totally eliminated in the USA. In the UK manufacturers have been forced to reduce the trans fat content of their products and some major supermarkets are now claiming that their own-brand products are totally free from trans fats.

Margarine, in its various forms, has been eaten, for over 40 years by countless millions of people thinking it was an integral part of their 'healthy eating plan'. In fact, it was highly toxic and a major cause of coronary artery disease,[47] and therefore much less healthy than the butter that they had denied themselves.

The cereal alternative

In contrast to traditional breakfasts high in fat and protein, the original cereals were initially almost totally devoid of vitamins, especially B vitamins. These are essential in the prevention of many conditions, including coronary artery disease via the homocysteine pathway as described in the last chapter. As early as 1968 the well-known American food campaigner, Robert Chote, famously pointed out on a CBS television programme that 'most cereal breakfasts [at that time] contain virtually no more nutritional content than the cardboard box they come in'. He described these products as 'empty calories', a term still in use today.

Eventually the cereal manufacturers agreed to add specific B vitamins, especially the ones identified with the homocysteine phenomenon. Later on, various whole-grain products appeared in response to public demand for healthier food.

The sugar content in the UK still remained a problem. In 2006 the broadcasting watchdog, OfCOM, judged that many cereals contained far too much sugar, and as a result of that they were no longer allowed to advertise on television when young children were watching. At last this official body had woken up to the dangers of refined sugar.

Cigarette smoking

There is an interesting connection between cigarette smoking and sugar in that in all British and American cigarettes, sugar, rum and flavourings are added in the curing process. This may possibly add to the addictive properties of cigarette smoke as well as the taste of the cigarette.

Many years ago, in my book entitled *Avoidable Death*, I concluded that cigarette smoking was, at that time, killing 300 people each day in England and Wales. This figure was confirmed by many sources a few years later. I was the first person, in a popular book, to argue that the 70% increase in coronary thrombosis in cigarette smokers was much more important than the 1080% increase in lung cancer. To increase the incidence of coronary thrombosis, a common disease in any case, had a much greater impact on overall mortality than the lung cancer figures. Lung cancer is a relatively rare condition in non-smokers.

The peak of the coronary epidemic in the UK was around 1965–70. At that time, 54% of the British population were smokers, smoking an average of 20 cigarettes a day. By 2008 the proportion of the population smoking had dropped to 21%, which of course meant that 33% of the population had stopped smoking. This reduction has been one of the most successful public health measures of all time, and has had a major influence on cardiac mortality.

So what has caused the reduction in coronary artery disease?

I have no doubt that 33% of the population in England and Wales ceasing to smoke has been the main reason for the reduction in death from heart disease between 1970 and 2010. In fact, this reduction should have been greater considering the millions of people who stopped. Coronary artery disease is still the leading cause of death, but if the cholesterol theory had been correct it should have virtually disappeared by now. Of course, as I pointed out in chapter 9, not one study looking at reducing dietary cholesterol has shown any reduction in coronary mortality. In any responsible scientific environment, there should have been considerable questioning as to why so little further progress has been made despite so many people being on low-fat diets.

Where there has been undoubted progress is in the development and acceptance of the role homocysteine plays in heart disease. Although it has been frequently mentioned in newspapers and magazines it has not, as yet, made very much impact on the general public. I have found it difficult to ascertain how many cardiologists and GPs are prescribing B vitamins to treat this cause of coronary artery disease.

Meanwhile, eminent physicians have continued to research the role of refined sugar and subsequent hyperinsulinaemia as *the* prime cause of type II diabetes and a major cause of coronary artery disease. Scientifically the evidence could hardly be stronger, but in America the official reports of the National Institute of Health and the American Heart Association remain wedded to the cholesterol/heart disease dogma. It seems to me that in the USA, at least, there is a determination to fight any suggestion that sugar is involved in any medical condition whatsoever despite overwhelming evidence that it is.

Chapter summary

- I am sure, for all the reasons I have described, that the toxic element in the diets of 'civilised' countries is refined carbohydrates, and if we went back to eating the unrefined versions we would all soon be much healthier and significantly slimmer.
- Man has made both cigarettes and refined carbohydrates. Cigarettes, as well as being responsible for 90% of all cases of lung cancer, are also a major contributor to coronary

artery disease. Refined carbohydrates lead to obesity, type II diabetes and a substantial proportion of coronary artery disease.

- Man blamed cholesterol instead of his own mistakes. Avoiding fat and promoting refined carbohydrates has trebled obesity levels.

Chapter 13

Does exercise help in weight management?

To many, at one time myself included, the old adage that if you are putting on weight all you need to do is eat less and exercise more seems eminently plausible. Since becoming involved with allergy and nutritional medicine I have come to realise that this is completely untrue. I've known for many years that you would have to run for 35 miles to burn 3500 calories and thereby one pound of fat. However, I used to think that heavy exercise must increase our metabolic rate and that increase would continue for many hours after the exercise was finished. It does in fact continue for a few hours, but not many.

Throughout my life I have been an enthusiast for sporting exercise, but I have always felt that this should be enjoyable. Putting on a tracksuit and pounding the streets, especially in a bleak British winter, does not come into that category for me. I take my hat off to the few that do it.

For years I advised those patients with a tendency to weight gain to take as much exercise as possible. As time passed I became less enthusiastic as no matter how hard my patients tried to follow my advice it made little difference.

In chapter 2, I discussed the adverse effects of low-calorie diets. It was thought by many that if exercise were incorporated with low-calorie diets they would be even more effective. This turned out not to be the case. In 22 studies,[48] the results of which were pooled together, patients were restricted to a diet of less than 1000 calories a day and at the same time were made to undertake heavy exercise. The combined results showed that, surprisingly, there was no overall weight loss achieved at all. This is the regime that many people have endured and still are enduring, while in most cases any initial loss is short-lived and weight steadily increases thereafter.

In another study,[49] women consumed a liquid diet supplying only 522 calories per day whilst partaking in weight training and endurance exercise. There was no improvement in their metabolism and in fact resting metabolic rate fell 7–12% in all of those involved.

I emphasise that all kinds of exercise programmes have been studied, including aerobic and anaerobic exercise, resistance training, combination approaches and long distance walking and jogging programmes. There is no doubt that exercise is good for your health and keeps your muscles well toned, making you look better, but as a tool simply for losing weight it doesn't work.

Case History: Helene J (aged 36)

Helene was an aerobics instructor in Hollywood in the 1960s and was involved with Jane Fonda in her famous exercise video in which the phrase 'going for the burn' originated. She later moved to England and set up an exercise studio. She specialised in two-hour sessions of high-speed 'step' classes to rock music. She described her clients as the crème-de-la-crème of exercise fanatics. She did these classes six days a week.

When she first arrived in England her weight was ideal, but despite all her exercise she had gained 12 lb (5.5 kg) by the time she came to see me. After the first seven days of my elimination diet she had lost 7 lb (3 kg) and several minor symptoms, and by the end of week four she had lost all 12 lb. By taking neutralisation for the four foods identified as problematic, she was able to continue eating normally while staying her ideal weight. Clearly you cannot exercise away a food sensitivity problem.

Exercise and coronary thrombosis

Data from the nurses health study[50] mentioned in chapter 9 has shown that brisk walking for one hour a day for four or more days a week lowered the risk of coronary thrombosis by 30-40%. This was a huge study based on 72,500 female nurses aged 40–65 years old. Brisk walking seems to be the safest and most reliable form of exercise, particularly for people over the age of 50.

Conclusion

I must emphasise that there is no doubt whatsoever that moderate exercise is a must for your general physical and mental health. It has major health benefits such as the cardiovascular effect mentioned above, and helps in reducing the amount of insulin produced by stimulating a more efficient use of glucose. Other additional benefits include increased muscle mass, better muscle definition and improved posture – all of which help you to look better as well as feel better. Many people note that they sleep better after exercise too.

Although a big fan of exercise myself, especially racquet sports, clinical experience over the years has left me disappointed at how little it appears to help my patients to lose weight. Clinical studies have borne out my observations. While I would encourage you to take up or continue with an exercise regime, I would also like you to realise it will not make a major contribution to your weight loss.

Chapter 14

A step-by-step programme to sort out your own weight problems

Your personal weight problems may have more than one cause. Having read the previous chapters you will have already formed an idea as to the areas you may need to tackle. This chapter will help you plan your approach systematically.

If you have been on a calorie-controlled diet recently you should first spend around three weeks on a diet of good quality food with no calorie restriction to **combat the low metabolic rate and increased insulation associated with calorie restriction**, as described in chapter 2. This diet can include the following foods which may, in the short term, lead initially to some weight gain as your body adjusts to the higher calorific intake:

- All meats, including lamb, beef, pork, chicken, duck and ham
- All fish including salmon, cod, trout, skate and all shell-fish
- Grains such as wholemeal bread, rye, oats, barley
- Whole grain rice
- All vegetables including potatoes (not chips)
- All salads (not pasta)
- Eggs
- Butter, milk, cheese, yoghurt (all full fat)
- All pulses, including beans and peas
- All fruits (not fruit juice)

By way of contrast, the following foods should be avoided:
- Refined carbohydrates including:
    - o   Sugar
    - o   White bread
    - o   Cakes
    - o   Biscuits
    - o   Pizza
    - o   Pasta (white)
    - o   Breakfastcereals(exceptporridgeoatsandshredded wheat)
    - o   Confectionary
    - o   Desserts
    - o   Ice cream
    - o   Most chocolate (apart from sugar-free)
    - o   Beer
    - o   Soft drinks containing sugar
    - o   White rice
- Any food which states on the label it is 'low fat/fat free'

Complex carbohydrates lead to a slow release of energy because it takes time to break them down to a simpler substance like glucose. Thus you should, by following the above regime, slowly reverse the processes leading to increased insulation and decreased metabolism. Often in the first week or so of this diet there is a slight weight gain followed by a slow decrease in weight.

After the three weeks on this diet (or straight away if you have not been on a calorie-controlled diet recently) you are ready to start the elimination diet.

As I have emphasised before, I think everyone should start addressing their weight problem with **the elimination diet** (chapter 5), as food sensitivity is by far the most common cause of weight problems. Furthermore, it only takes seven days to reach a positive or negative conclusion. If you have lost no weight by day seven you should abandon the elimination diet.

This diet allows 40 foods, but only these foods (with not even a sip or taste of anything else), which share just one virtue: they all have a very low risk of being the cause of a food sensitivity. They can all be eaten in any quantity. People who cannot lose weight on a 1000 calorie diet, will commonly lose substantial weight on this diet despite eating over 2500 calories a day.

This diet is also not a low-carbohydrate diet as it contains several high-carbohydrate vegetables, including sweet potatoes, parsnips, swedes and lentils. In addition, it also contains high-carbohydrate fruits.

The greatest feature of this diet is that weight loss (and loss of symptoms, if any) will happen very quickly. For example, someone who is 25 lb (11.5 kg) overweight can lose 8 lb (3.5 kg) or more in the first seven days. Most people will experience 'withdrawal symptoms' starting on the evening of the first day and lasting for over three days. These symptoms are not caused by the foods you are eating, but a reaction to what you are not eating in a similar, but much milder way, to an alcoholic coming off drink. After the sixth/seventh day you should feel much brighter than usual. If you do feel rough at first, don't worry as it is a very good sign because it indicates that you do indeed have a food sensitivity and are doing the right thing. If you have absolutely no symptoms before starting the diet it is unlikely you will have any withdrawal symptoms but nevertheless should still lose weight. If you find you have lost weight on stage one, then progress onto the second and third stages of the diet.

If you have not lost a reasonable amount of weight by the end of week one then you have to consider other possible causes of weight gain: **underactive thyroid, the yeast syndrome, and insulin resistance.** You can begin by looking at the two questionnaires that follow to see if they highlight one of those problems for you.

Questionnaires

1. *To identify a problem with the yeast syndrome*

Women are more likely than men to have this problem, probably because of their complex hormone systems; there is a distinct link between yeast hypersensitivity and 'hormonal'-type symptomatology. This section of the questionnaire is divided into two parts: firstly the predisposing factors, and secondly the consequences.

Predisposing factors

1. Have you taken more than one course of antibiotics in the last five years? Or, alternatively, have you taken antibiotics at any time in your life for more than two months, as in treatment for acne or long-term infections?	Point Score 10 30
2. Do you live in a damp mouldy house with visible mould on the walls and also, for example, around the bottom of windows?	10
3. Do you eat a lot of sugar? Please note that non-diet soft drinks, such as colas, may have more than five teaspoons of sugar in each can. Cakes, biscuits, ice creams, yogurts, sweets, chocolate, etc, all contain a lot of sugar. Moderate consumption Large consumption	10 15
4. Do you consume a lot of yeasty products, such as alcohol (especially beer, wine and champagne rather than spirits), bread, cheese, mushrooms, vinegar, Marmite? Moderate consumption Large consumption	5 10
5. Do you suffer from diabetes?	10

6. Steroids: Have you taken steroids such as cortisone or prednisalone by mouth: For up to four weeks? For more than four weeks?	 5 10
Women only, for obvious reasons!	
7. Have you been pregnant: Once? Two or more times?	 3 5
8. Have you taken the contraceptive pill: For up to six months? For up to two years? For more than two years?	 5 10 15
9. Have you taken hormone replacement therapy in tablet form: For a few months? For over one year?	 5 10

The maximum score in this section is 85 for men and 115 for women.

Consequences

	Point Score
1. Do you suffer from excessive wind and bloating of the abdomen, the bloating at times looking like early pregnancy?	 30
2. Do you have indigestion and/or heart-burn?	10
3. Do you suffer from thrush? That is vag-inal or oral thrush in women and penile or oral thrush in men: Rarely? Frequently?	 10 30
4. Do you suffer from bowel irregularity, either: Constipation? Or diarrhoea? Or constipation alternating with diar-rhoea?	 30 5 5

5. Do you notice irritation around your anus Rarely? Frequently?	 5 10
6. Do you suffer from athlete's foot, ring-worm, jock itch, or other long-term fungal infection of the skin or nails: Occasionally? Frequently? Continuously?	 5 15 20
7. If you are under 50, do you have problems with memory and/or con-centration?	 20
8. Do you crave sugary food?	10
9. Are you prone to suffering from cysti-tis or frequency of urination with some degree of 'burning'? In addition, if you have urine cultures, do they usually prove negative?	 10 15
10. Does alcohol upset you, even if taken in small quantities?	 10
11. Are you worse when the weather is damp?	 10
12. Do you have a loss of sexual desire or impotence?	 10
13. Do you suffer from psoriasis?	10
14. Do you have problems with poor co-ordination?	 10
15. Are you sensitive to chemical odours, such as petrol fumes, diesel fumes, paint fumes, perfumes etc?	 10

Women only	
16. Did the contraceptive pill upset you in any way when you first took it, e.g. headache, depression or weight gain?	10
17. Did hormone replacement therapy taken by mouth have similar adverse effects?	10
18. Do you feel distinctly worse premenstrually, e.g. with depression, tension, water retention, breast tenderness and/or headaches?	10
19. Do you suffer from endometriosis, polycystic ovaries or infertility?	5

What makes the diagnosis of the yeast syndrome even more likely is that the 'consequences' (the last 19 symptoms) are noticeably worse after contact with the 'predisposing factors'. An obvious example would be if you had a flare-up of any symptoms or your weight increased noticeably after a course of antibiotics. If the score for the 'predisposing factors' and the 'consequences' are added together the maximum score for women would be 345 whereas for men it would be 285. In women, any score of less than 60 (men less than 50) would suggest that a yeast problem is unlikely to be a factor in their weight problems. In both sexes, scores of over a 100 make the problem likely. In any woman, a score of over 180, or in a man, a score of over 140, would make the diagnosis a certainty. However, even if the score is very high, while it does mean you have a problem with yeast, it does not necessarily mean that this is the whole cause of your weight problems.

2. To identify hypothyroidism

This condition is caused by a deficiency of thyroid hormones as described in chapter 8.

	Point score
1. Fatigue Mild Severe	5 10
2. Slow pulse rate – 60 beats per minute or less	15
3. Low temperature Less than 35.8° C (96.4° F) when measured with the thermometer under the armpit first thing in the morning before rising	20
4. Swelling of thyroid gland This is found at the front of the neck and the swelling is known as a goitre	40
5. Thinning of outer third of eyebrows	20
6. Small little finger If your little finger does not reach the last knuckle of the next finger (Possibly a genetic pre-disposition)	10

The highest possible score is 115. Any score above 50 suggests you have hypothyroidism. This condition has nothing to do with your diet so no form of dietary change will improve it. You must therefore consult a doctor who specialises in this subject.

3. To identify a problem with high insulin levels (hyperinsulinaemia)

If you are still significantly overweight despite trying to address food sensitivity and a yeast problem and the questionnaire doesn't suggest you might have a thyroid problem, then hyperinsulinaemia is highly likely. If this is the case there is nothing to stop you from trying a low-carbohydrate diet, such as the ones outlined in chapter 10. If you want definitive proof, then there are blood tests available:

- Glucose tolerance test – This involves first taking a blood sample after you have fasted, usually overnight to see what your normal level is. You are then asked to swallow a measured dose of glucose. Blood samples are then taken at half-hourly intervals for 2.5 hours. Certainly a result that says you are pre-diabetic or diabetic is concrete proof.
- Serum insulin – If this result is higher than the normal range this again is definite proof of poorly functioning carbohydrate metabolism.

The best treatment for hyperinsulinaemia, in my opinion, is the low-carbohydrate diet described by Dr Robert Atkins in his book *Dr Atkins' New Diet Revolution*. To do the diet properly you will need to buy this book. If you have already sorted out any food sensitivity problems, then you shouldn't run into the complications that can occur with this diet that I described in chapter 10.

A substantial weight loss in the first two weeks of this diet (the induction phase) accompanied by the presence of ketones in the urine confirms the diagnosis of hyperinsulinaemia. You should then follow the other stages in the book, and will doubtless continue to lose weight, hopefully down to your ideal weight.

When you have reached the higher carbohydrate stages of the Atkins diet, the glycaemic index of various foods can be very helpful, particularly when selecting foods to stay within your carbohydrate allowance at each subsequent phase (chapter 10). I emphasise that at all times, no matter what the Atkins book says, DO NOT eat a food to which you have found you are sensitive.

Chapter 15

In a nutshell ...

There can be few greater causes of unhappiness than the modern epidemic of weight problems and clinical obesity that has spread through much of the world, but especially the English-speaking countries. However happy a marriage, however delightful a lifestyle, if a person is substantially overweight, s/he may well be very unhappy and frustrated, particularly if s/he was slim only a few years before. Successfully losing weight is currently seen as hugely challenging as it is impossible to stay slim for the long term on a low-fat diet, but really it is all very simple. The six secrets of successful weight loss are:

ONE: Avoid low-calorie diets

Part of the frustration most people encounter who embark on low-calorie diets is that if they follow them religiously they do lose weight for a few weeks, but then it all goes wrong. Initial weight loss is followed by what is called 'stabilisation', when no further weight is lost despite strict adherence to the diet. After this, the weight often starts creeping back again, although there has been no deviation from the diet. Millions of people have noticed this frustrating phenomenon.

What has happened is that two weight conserving mechanisms have clicked in, triggered by the body interpreting low-calorie dieting as a form of starvation. These mechanisms, which were essential to our Stone Age ancestors, who often faced periods of starvation, are a reduction in metabolic rate and an increase in the body's insulation. The details are described in chapter 2. Repeated attempts at low-calorie dieting can result in more and more insulation and a lower and lower metabolic rate. Thus repeated attempts at low-calorie dieting can make it an effective way of actually gaining weight. As one book stated, 'Dieting can make you fat'.

To be clear, I totally agree that day-to-day variations in weight can relate in most overweight people to variations in excess calorie consumption. However, when you decide to restrict your calorie consumption severely over a period of several weeks, your body's anti-starvation mechanisms will take over and thwart the whole process.

TWO: Avoid low fat diets

Low-fat diets were originally advocated as a result of the theory that dietary cholesterol was somehow implicated in heart disease. In 1977 Senator George McGovern's *Dietary Goals for Americans* was published. In the next few years several other eminent bodies declared that dietary cholesterol was unhealthy and that all Americans should significantly reduce consumption of animal fat/cholesterol. At the same time Americans were advised to increase consumption of carbohydrates. This was aimed at reducing coronary artery disease. Shortly afterwards the same advice was given to the British. Before this many doctors and books had recommended decreasing carbohydrates for people with weight problems. Thus the new low-fat advice was the complete opposite of all previous advice. At no time in modern medical history had medical organisations suggested such major changes to the diet of their people on such minimal evidence, as I demonstrate in chapter 9.

Throughout most of the 1960s and 1970s approximately 8% of the British population and 12-13% of the American population were categorised as clinically obese. This figure had been fairly constant throughout those two decades. By 1980, low-fat diets had become well established on both sides of the Atlantic; a mere 25 years later the obesity rates in both countries had trebled.

In total contrast, the French eat by far the highest fat and lowest refined sugar diet in mainland Europe. Not only are the French the slimmest nation in Europe, but they have a very low rate of coronary artery disease compared to the UK and USA.

One of the problems with low-fat diets is that many people don't realise just how fattening they can be. Removing fat from the diet leads to eating more carbohydrates (the fat has to be replaced by something), which in turn leads to a higher risk of weight gain, diabetes and heart disease – the very thing that the majority of people were trying to avoid in the first place with the low-fat diet.

Surely a low fat diet is good for my heart?

The answer to that is an emphatic NO and I have devoted four whole chapters to explaining in detail why this is the case. Briefly, it came about because of the theory that eating cholesterol was a significant cause of coronary artery disease. However, this has been proved wrong in a very spectacular way, and we now have a much better idea of what really is to blame, as I go on to summarise later in this chapter (see 'The rise and fall of the cholesterol theory').

THREE: Sort out your food sensitivities

When I look at the jigsaw puzzle of all of the factors causing the huge epidemic of weight gain, the largest part of it is, in my experience, each person's individual food sensitivities, yet in all the diet books I have perused I have seen this mentioned only once. In over 30 years in clinical practice, tackling food sensitivities has been the approach that has worked time and again for patient after patient. The five people described in chapter 3 are typical of the many patients I used to see day after day. Medical colleagues working in the same area report very similar results.

Thirty-four years ago I started investigating the role of food sensitivity as a cause of illness. In the UK I was the first to devise a dietary strategy that could be used easily on an outpatient basis (as opposed to in a hospital setting). Other doctors also used my diet. Over the years, as my experience increased, I was able to refine the diet. My most up-to-date version is set out in chapter 5.

It must be emphasised that food sensitivities can develop at any time in your life, and the onset of weight gain (or symptoms) can be insidious. Sometimes the development of one or more food sensitivity can follow a viral infection, especially glandular fever or a severe dose of flu.

Elimination diets are very useful for identifying food sensitivities responsible for conditions such as migraine, headaches, depression, chronic fatigue, irritable bowel syndrome, Crohn's disease, eczema, urticaria and rheumatoid arthritis. Weight problems by themselves (or in addition to a variety of symptoms) are no exception. Somewhere between 70% and 80% of all the people who embarked on my elimination diet lost all or a substantial part of their excess weight.

Very few people who have sensitivities to everyday foods such as wheat, corn, milk, yeast and eggs, have the slightest inkling that their problems are caused by such apparently benign foods. This is because of a phenomenon called 'masking' which ensures that the adverse effects of the offending foods remain completely hidden. This is described in detail in chapter 4.

The practical importance of this masking is that a high proportion of people who are food sensitive will have a withdrawal reaction, starting, usually, late on the first day of the diet, and often lasting three or four days. The exciting thing is that many people will emerge from the first few days feeling better than they have in years. If you only have weight problems and no symptoms at all, you will have no withdrawal symptoms whatsoever. However, a decent loss of weight by day seven will identify food sensitivity as the cause of your weight problems.

If you identify food sensitivity as the cause of your weight problems it is very good news, as the whole sorting-out procedure can be accomplished in six to eight weeks by following the next two stages of the diet as set out in chapter 5.

If all of your excess weight disappears on this procedure, then all you need to do is to avoid the foods that you now know you are sensitive to. However, if at the outset you have a lot of weight to lose you may find that you continue to lose weight slowly and gradually over the next few months. If avoiding certain foods appears to be too difficult you may like to consider contacting a clinic that specialises in desensitising people to their individual food sensitivities (see appendix II). Details of the pros and cons of using desensitisation are discussed in chapter 6.

By the end of the diet all the work has been done. By avoiding the foods you now know to be problematic you may continue to lose weight slowly and gradually over the next few months. If the weight loss grinds to a halt and you would like ultimately to lose more then you will need to consider the other causes of weight problems that I have outlined. Completing the question-naires in chapter 14 should give you guidance as to which area to explore next.

FOUR: Treat the yeast syndrome if indicated

'Endotoxins' excreted by an overgrowth of yeasts in the gut can have an adverse effect on your weight-regulating mechanisms in a similar way to food sensitivities. A high consumption of re-fined sugar, yeasts in foods (e.g. bread) and alcohol, plus taking antibiotics and/or the contraceptive pill can all encourage this situation to occur. These yeast problems can also lead to recurring vaginal thrush, psoriasis, fungal types of eczema, urticaria (hives), and poor memory and concentration levels. It is necessary to embark on a diet that is low in sugars and yeasts while taking anti-yeast medication or supplements.

The three phases of the anti-yeast diet and various anti-yeast medications and supplements are described in chapter 7. The yeast syndrome has enormous importance as the fungal form of certain yeasts is known to penetrate the lining of the intestines leading to increased permeability and what is known as 'leaky gut syndrome'.

Many doctors who work in this field think that this situation leads to the development of food sensitivity and as such could hardly be more important.

FIVE: Reduce high levels of insulin (hyperinsulinaemia) if suspected

'Hyperinsulinaemia' means that your pancreas is producing unduly high levels of insulin. This is caused solely by regularly eating high amounts of carbohydrates, especially refined carbohydrates. High levels of insulin in the blood convert refined carbohydrates to fat. Insulin is known as the 'fattening hormone'. This is explained in detail in chapter 10. In particular, anyone with a positive glucose tolerance test should go onto a low-carbohydrate diet after sorting out any food sensitivities.

People who are very overweight often have a distinct problem with high levels of insulin. The logical response to this problem is to follow a low-carbohydrate diet.

Low-carbohydrate diets were first advocated in 1862 with the publication of the Banting diet. This and other low-carbohydrate diets were used by doctors for over 100 years with fairly good results. They were certainly much more effective than low-calorie or low-fat diets.

Some doctors have claimed that high levels of insulin are the only cause of weight problems, but I am certain from all of my years of clinical experience that food sensitivity is more common.

There are two main types of low-carbohydrate diet:

- **Atkins-type diets**: These initially limit carbohydrates to 20 grams daily for two weeks, with the carbohydrates used being derived from vegetables and salads. Fat and protein are unlimited. This is later expanded to 40 grams of carbohydrates daily, and later still, up to 60 grams. *Dr Atkins' Diet Revolution* is by far the biggest selling diet book in history. I usually suggest this option to people with hyperinsulinaemia after they have sorted out any food sensitivities

- **Low-glycaemic index (GI) diets**: The glycaemic index is a ranking of how fast foods are absorbed into the bloodstream. Low-GI diets utilise many more carbohydrates, but only those that are absorbed more slowly. It is my experience that these diets by themselves are not as dramatically effective as the first (induction) phase of the Atkins diet. Having said that, low-GI diets are much better than low-calorie or low-fat diets. I have listed the GI ratings of most commonly eaten foods in chapter 10. If you continue on the Atkins diet until the maintenance phase when carbohydrates are included in greater quantities, then the glycaemic index becomes a very useful tool.

SIX: Have low thyroid levels (hypothyroidism) investigated

Low levels of thyroxin, the hormone produced by your thyroid gland, have been known for many decades to be a cause of weight gain. This condition has nothing to do with diets and treatment relies entirely on hormone testing and replacement, when necessary, and so has to be carried out by a medical specialist.

The rise and fall of the cholesterol theory

Chapters 9 to 13 explain why the cholesterol theory is wrong and why eating a low-fat diet is so unhealthy. In the early days of the cholesterol theory there were a few 'facts' that appeared, at first, possibly to support it. These were:

- Force feeding rabbits with a high-cholesterol diet led to plaques in their arteries which were full of cholesterol. The fundamental flaw with this is, of course, that rabbits are herbivores and as such never eat animal fat. Consequently, they have no mechanisms for dealing with animal products. Later experiments with feeding meat-eating animals with high-cholesterol diets showed no adverse effect at all.

- The 'Seven Countries study', conducted by Dr Ancel Keyes, did show some correlation between countries that consumed high levels of animal fat and had high rates of coronary artery disease. However, when all 20 countries that had adequate statistics available were included (instead of just selecting seven of them) there was no correlation at all. These days such manipulation of research statistics would be regarded as research fraud.

- The early reports from the famous Framingham study noted that people with a high level of cholesterol in their blood had slightly higher rates of coronary artery disease and mortality. After the study had continued for longer it was found that the earlier findings were not substantiated.

- Initially a study in Helsinki appeared to show a decreased death rate from coronary artery disease in patients on low-saturated-fat diets. After another 10 years of study the cardiac mortality in the low-fat dieters had doubled compared with the controls who ate normally.

So there was, initially, some suggestion that the theory was correct, but in the long run the evidence did not hold up at all.

There have now been, worldwide, around 30 studies involving large populations of normal healthy people who have been put on low-fat diets and compared with equal numbers of people eating each country's usual diet. Some of these studies have shown a reduction in serum cholesterol levels on those on low-fat diets. These were reported as a triumph, and this helped to keep the cholesterol theory alive in some people's minds. However, not one study showed a decrease in mortality from coronary thrombosis in the low-fat diet groups, and a number of studies showed a distinct increase in coronary artery mortality. Not one study established a causal relationship between eating high-saturated-fat diets and coronary artery mortality.

As each study was reported there was much speculation in newspapers as well as medical journals about the 'death of the low-fat diet myth'. At one time the *Sunday Times* devoted an entire colour supplement to this topic and asked the question 'Is It All a Big Fat Lie?'

After spending 11 years conducting studies to write a report supporting the cholesterol theory, the USA's Surgeon General abandoned the project. This report remains unpublished, and all one or the organisers had to say was to admit that the work did not confirm the validity of the theory.

At one time the discovery and use of statin drugs appeared to have rescued the cholesterol theory. Statin drugs do reduce cholesterol and have some effect in reducing mortality from coronary artery disease. However, their beneficial effect is thought to be related to reducing fibrinogen, a clotting agent in the blood, and not to their cholesterol-lowering effect.

It is vital that you understand that the cholesterol theory is totally wrong. Low-fat diets are not a healthy option, and are the major reason why there has been such an explosion in obesity and type II diabetes since 1980.

If the public are to continue to be misled by the cholesterol theory, obesity will continue to rise. There is no evidence that dietary advice generated from the cholesterol theory has prevented even one death. There is, however, plenty of evidence that it has not prevented any deaths from coronary artery disease, or any other disease. Some studies have even shown an increased death rate in people on low-cholesterol diets.

What the 'experts' now say

- Dr Ancel Keyes, author of the 'Seven Countries study and the main protagonist of the 'cholesterol theory', stated in 1997: 'There is no connection whatsoever between cholesterol in food, and cholesterol in the blood, and we have known that all along. Cholesterol in the diet does not matter at all unless you happen to be a chicken or a rabbit.'
- Dr William Castelli, the then Director of the prestigious Framingham study, that had been continuing for 50 years, said in 1998: 'The more saturated fat one ate, the more cholesterol one ate, the more calories one ate, the lower the person's serum cholesterol. We also found that people who ate the most cholesterol and ate the most calories weighed the least and were the most physically active.'
- Dr George Mann, who was an earlier Director of the Framingham Study, stated: 'The diet/heart hypothesis has been repeatedly shown to be wrong, and yet for complicated reasons of pride, profit and prejudice the hypothesis continues to be exploited by scientists' fund-raising enterprises, food companies and even governmental agencies. The public is being deceived by the greatest health scam of the century.'

Historical evidence that refined carbohydrates are the real culprits

We have eaten meat, fish, fruit and vegetables for over two million years. Ten thousand years ago we started to eat wheat, corn and other whole grains. The keeping of sheep and herds of cattle in order to provide a regular supply of meat and milk started several thousand years before the birth of Christ. The consumption of eggs started at about the same time. Thus we have eaten meat for millions of years and milk and eggs for thousands of years. In the 1970s we were told that at the beginning of the 20th century all of a sudden these foods had started to attack us and within a few decades were the cause of death of around 40% of the population in the western world. This is so utterly preposterous that I have been never been able to take the cholesterol theory seriously.

So what was the dietary change that caused coronary thrombosis? There was, in my opinion, only one possibility, and that was refined carbohydrates. In all fairness, unrefined and refined carbohydrates were initially included under one heading in government statistics. This was why it did not become obvious to begin with. Later, the statistics were altered and the descriptions 'refined carbohydrates', and 'unrefined carbohydrates' were put under separate headings. The production of refined sugar and flour started around 1850–70. Obesity started to become much more common within a few years. Type II diabetes was first diagnosed in the 1870s. Coronary artery disease followed in 1912.

The refining process strips sugar and wholemeal flour of most of their naturally occurring nutrients. In the case of sugar, 98% of the nutrient chromium is lost. Chromium is essential for the metabolic pathway that processes sugar after you have eaten it. Thus the refining of sugar exerts its adverse effects from its high speed of absorption and by the loss of chromium. I have described how this leads to hyperinsulinaemia, insulin resistance, type II diabetes and coronary thrombosis in chapter 11. High levels of insulin are a potent cause of weight problems which can be addressed by an Atkins-type low-carbohydrate diet.

Refining wholemeal flour also leads to some loss of chromium, but the main loss is of various B vitamins. Very soon after refined flour became available, beri beri, caused by vitamin B_1 deficiency, and pellagra, caused by vitamin B_3 deficiency, led to epidemics, killing millions of people until the situation was corrected.

In the last few decades, Dr Kilmer McCully recognised that deficiencies in vitamins B_6, B_{12} and folic acid were leading to increases in the blood levels of the amino acid 'homocysteine'. This is now recognised as a major cause of coronary artery disease, strokes and several other medical conditions. You may have noticed that I use the word 'cause', as administration of these B vitamins has been shown in major clinical studies to reverse cardiac symptoms and extend life expectancy by around eight years in people with high levels of homocysteine in their blood stream. Had these inexpensive B vitamins been an expensive drug everyone would have known about homocysteine for several years. However, this homocysteine treatment is now accepted and is described in standard cardiology textbooks.

The evidence shows, in my view, that there are four distinct pathways in the production of coronary disease:
- Cigarette smoking – now totally proven.
- High levels of homocysteine, which the body cannot metabolise and remove without the presence of vitamins B_6, B_{12} and folic acid.
- Chromium deficiency, which is caused by the consumption of refined sugar.
- Trans fatty acids, found in margarine and many processed foods, which are now established as a distinct cause of coronary thrombosis. They have been completely banned in some countries and others are planning to follow suit.[47]

What I find so utterly compelling about the refined carbo-hydrate story is that the same sequence of events that I have described occurred when certain primitive peoples were intro-duced to the same refined carbohydrates, around 50 years later – that is, after a few years, obesity was observed followed by diabetes and later coronary artery disease.

So what is the current situation regarding weight/health?

The current weight/health situation can be summarised by the following:

- Weight problems and clinical obesity are continuing to increase, and are expected to do so for many years.
- Diabetes is increasing rapidly, with the last five years showing a steeper rise. This situation is made even worse by the way it is treated.
- In the USA the decline in the death rate from coronary artery disease stopped in the 1990s and has now started to climb again, as discovered by a major study of post mortem results.[51]
- The increase in the death rate from coronary artery disease is attributed to the rise in diabetes and obesity, but these conditions are being accentuated by the same low-fat/high-carbohydrate diets that I have been talking about throughout this book.

There has been little research into the causes of weight gain or obesity in the past. Now the medical profession appears to have largely given up researching what is the greatest medical and social problem of our age.

A lot of the problems in medicine as a whole are related to the adverse influence of the pharmaceutical and food industries. There is no doubt that money can buy both science and medical attitudes. If you are interested in looking at how this situation has arisen then there are a number of books on the market. I would particularly recommend three, which are *Trick and Treat* by Barry Groves, *The Diet Delusion* by Gary Taubes and *Malignant Medical Myths* by Professor Joel Kauffman.

Chapter summary

- Many people suffer, usually unknowingly, from food sensitivities. These sensitivities are generally to commonly eaten foods, such as wheat, corn, milk, eggs, yeast and cane sugar. Most people usually eat these foods on a daily basis. In over 70% of people, identifying and avoiding the foods that cause sensitivities can improve or totally eradicate their weight problems.
- Approximately a quarter of the adult population, especially women, are affected at some time in their lives, by an excess of yeasts in the gut. The toxins from these can disturb your weight-regulating mechanisms.
- Having constantly high levels of the hormone insulin (a condition called hyperinsulinaemia) is a result of high consumption of refined carbohydrates – principally, sugar and flour. These are, of course found in many everyday foods such as most breakfast cereals, cakes, biscuits, sweetened drinks and white breads. Insulin converts these refined carbohydrates into fat.
- Low-fat diets inevitably increase the consumption of refined carbohydrates, making hyperinsulinaemia and the yeast problem worse. Diets that are low in fat make feeling full more difficult, because your appetite is not satisfied.
- Countries that eat low-fat/high-carbohydrates diets are the fattest in the world and also have the highest incidence of diabetes and coronary artery disease. In countries

where people have been strongly encouraged to reduce fat in their diet, obesity has trebled.

- Low-calorie diets usually only work for a few weeks as they cause a lowering of the metabolism and encourage the laying down of fat to increase insulation – responses that served our Stone Age ancestors well at times of food shortage.

- Although excellent for general health, strenuous exercise has relatively little benefit as a method of losing weight. Weight gain results from a genuine metabolic imbalance that needs to be dealt with first by addressing its root causes.

Appendix I

Foods containing wheat, corn, milk, yeast and soy

I am now including some helpful (I hope) lists of foods containing wheat, corn, milk, yeast and soy. Foods containing some of these five ingredients are the most difficult to avoid. Some of my patients have opted for desensitisation therapy (see chapter 6) after seeing these lists, but it is in fact possible to eat well avoiding all these manufactured items. It does, however, mean sticking to a whole-food diet of simple meats, fowl, fish, fruit, vegetables, grains and nuts.

Foods containing wheat

Bread
Biscuits
Cereal-derived sauces
Cheese spreads containing
  cereal products as fillers
Chocolate (all except bitter
  chocolate)
Coffee substitutes
Commercial cakes
Crackers made from wheat
Commercial salad dressings
  made with wheat flour
Canned & frozen foods (some)
Flour
Gravies
Ice cream
Ice cream cones
Tortillas

Luncheon meats
Macaroni
Malt
Meat loaf
Meat or fish burgers
Noodles
Pastas
Oatmeal (some)
Ovaltine
Pastries & pies
Puddings
Pancake
Sausages
Soups thickened with wheat
  flour
Any sauce or gravy thickened
  with wheat flour
Spaghetti

Vermicelli
Various alcoholic drinks

Waffles
Most beers, whiskies and gins

Foods containing corn

Bacon (some)
Baking powders
Biscuits
Breads and pastries (some)
Cakes
Chocolate
Cough syrups
Canned peas
Coated rice
Dates (sweetened)
Frozen juices (some)
Gelatin desserts
Grape juice (some)
Hams (some)
Icing sugar
Instant teas (some)
Jellies
Margarine
Popcorn
Puddings
Sandwich spreads
Sundaes
Starch (cornflour)

Baking mixtures
Batters
Bleached wheat flour
Carbonated beverages (most)
Cheeses (some)
Cornflakes
Cream pies
Custards
Canned fruits (some)
Deep fat frying mixtures
Fruit juices (some)
Glucose products
Gravies
Ice cream
Instant coffee (some)
Jams
Milk in paper cartons
Peanut butter
Preserves
Salad dressings
Sauces
Sherbets
String beans – canned and Soups
   frozen (some)

Soya milks (some)
Sweeteners
Tortillas
Vegetables – canned and
   frozen (some)

Syrups
Sweets
Vanilla
Vinegar (some)

Most tablets, capsules, lozenges, suppositories

Alcohol:
   most beers
   gins
   cheap wines

whiskies
sherries
(See also page 76)

Foods containing milk or milk products

Au gratin foods
  (potatoes, beans)
Boiled salad dressings
Butter
Butter sauces
Candies
Chocolate or cocoa drinks
Cream
Cream sauces
Custards
Eggs, scrambled
Hamburger buns
Mashed potatoes
Margarine
Milk (condensed, dried,
  evaporated, powdered)
Mixes for:
  biscuits
  cakes
  doughnuts
  muffins
  pancakes
  pie crust
  puddings
  waffles

Baking powder biscuits
Baker's bread
Bologna
Buttermilk
Cakes
Cheese
Chowders
Creamed foods
Curd
Doughnuts
Gravy
Ice cream
Malted milk
Meat loaf
Omelettes
Quiche
Rarebits
Salad dressings
Soda crackers
Soufflés
Soups
Waffles
Whey
Yogurt

Foods containing yeast

1. Foods that contain yeast as an added ingredient

- Breads
- Biscuits
- Pastries
- Pretzels
- Hamburgers
- Rolls and buns, including hot-dog rolls
- Cakes and cake mix
- Flour enriched with yeast vitamins
- Milk fortified with vitamins from yeast
- Foods in dried breadcrumbs

2. Foods that contain yeast naturally

The following foods contain yeast or yeast–like substances because of their nature or the nature of their manufacture or preparation:

- Mushrooms, truffles and other edible fungi
- Cheeses of all kinds, including cottage cheese
- Buttermilk
- Various vinegars, such as apple, pear, grape, and distilled vinegar. These vinegars can also occur in mayonnaise, olives, pickles, sauerkraut, condiments, horseradish, French dressings, salad dressings, barbecue sauce, tomato sauce, chilli peppers, and mince pies
- All alcoholic drinks, including whiskies, gins, wines, brandy, rum, vodka, beer
- Malted products, including cereals, sweets, chocolates, and milk drinks which have been malted
- Citrus fruit drinks, either frozen or canned. Almost all commercial fruit juices contain yeast.

3. Vitamin supplements

Many vitamin products are derived from yeast or have their sources in yeast.

Foods containing soya beans

- Bakery goods – Soy bean flour containing only 1% of oil is now used by some bakeries in their dough mixtures for breads, rolls, cakes and pastries.
- Salad dressing – Many salad dressings and mayonnaises contain soya oil, but only state on the label that they contain vegetable oil.
- Meats – Pork sausage and luncheon meats may contain soya beans.
- Sweets – Soya flour is used in hard sweets. Lecithin is invariably derived from soya beans and is used in sweets to prevent drying out, and to emulsify the fats.
- Milk substitutes – Some bakers use soya milk instead of cows' milk.
- Ice cream
- Soups
- Vegetables – Fresh soya sprouts are served as a vegetable, especially in Chinese dishes.
- Soya nuts are roasted, salted and used instead of peanuts.
- Soya bean noodles, macaroni, and spaghetti
- Margarine and butter substitutes.

Appendix II

Where to get help

National bodies that can advise on finding an appropriate doctor

British Society of Ecological Medicine
Administrator
BSEM
c/o New Medicine Group
144 Harley Street
London W1G 7LE
thebsem@gmail.com

Thyroid UK
32 Darcy Road
St Osyth
Clacton-on-Sea
Essex CO16 8QF
Tel: +44 (0)1255 820407
www.thyroid.org.uk

American Academy of Environmental Medicine
There are several hundred doctors in the USA practising this form of medicine. Most are members of the American Academy of Environmental Medicine. These can be found by looking at their website, www.aaem. org under the heading of community resources/find an aaem member.

Prominent members of the British Society of Ecological Medicine

Professor J Brostoff
34 Fitzroy Avenue
London NW3 5NB
Tel: +44 (0)20 7435 7106

Dr Damien Downing
144 Harley Street
London W1G 7LE
Tel: +44 (0)20 7099 6003

Dr Charles Forsyth
Surrey: North Cottage
Dovers Green Road
Reigate RH2 8BU
Tel: +44 (0)1737 226338
Central London: Biolab Medical Unit
The Stone House
9 Weymouth Street
London W1W 6DB
Tel: +44 (0)20 7636 5905
Email: office@dr-forsyth.com
Website: www.dr-forsyth.com

Dr Nicola Hembry
Litfield House Medical Centre,
1 Litfield Place
Clifton Down
Bristol BS8 3LS
Tel: +44 (0)117 317 1460
Fax: +44 (0)117 973 3303,
Email: info@drhembry.com
Website: www.drhembry.com

Dr John Meldrum
Scotland: Mulberry House,

13 Inverleith Row
Edinburgh H3 5LS
Tel: +44 (0)1904 691591
York: Nutrition Associates,
Galtres House, Lysander Close
York YO3 4XB
Tel: +44 (0)1904 691591

Dr Sarah Myhill
Upper Weston, LLangunllo, Knighton
Powys LD7 1SL
Tel: +44 (0)1547 550611
Email: caroline@drmyhill.co.uk
Website www.drmyhill.co.uk

Dr Shideh Pouria
The Burghwood Clinic
34 Brighton Road, Banstead
Surrey SM7 1BS
Tel: +44 (0)1737 361177
Email: info@burghwoodclinic.co.uk
Website: www.burghwoodclinic.co.uk

Dr Michael Radcliffe
Sarum Road Hospital
Sarum Road, Winchester
Hampshire SO22 5HA
Tel: +44 (0)1962 844555

Addresses of recommended clinics offering desensitisation in the UK

The Burghwood Clinic
34 Brighton Road
Banstead
Surrey SM7 1BS
Tel: +44 (0)1737 361177
www.burghwoodclinic.co.uk

Dr Jean Munro
The Brakespear Hospital
Hertfordshire House
Wood Lane
Paradise Industrial Estate
Hemel Hempstead
Herts HP2 4FD
Tel: +44 (0)1442 261333
www.brakespearmedical.com

Dr Apelles Econs
Website: www.allergymedicaluk.com
Surrey: Marlborough House
68 High Street
Weybridge
Surrey KT13 8BL
Tel: +44 (0)1535 603966
Oxford: Raleigh Park Clinic
Raleigh Park Road
Oxford OX2 9AR
Tel: +44 (0)1932 820578
West Yorkshire: 41 Devonshire Street
Keighley
West Yorkshire BD21 2BH
Tel: +44 (0)1535 603966

Supplements

To lower homocysteine levels

Although you can take the individual vitamins separately (B_6, B_{12} and folic acid), I recommend taking a formulation specially designed for this purpose. However, there are others on the market which I am sure are fine I personally use *H Factors* by Higher Nature (www.highernature.co.uk).

Help with sugar metabolism

Take one chromium picolinate 200 µg per day. These supplements are usually very inexpensive and many makes are available in all good health food shops.

For medical professionals

Laboratories for nutritional assays in the UK

Biolab Medical Unit
The Stone House
9 Weymouth Street
London W1W 6DB
Tel: +44 (0)20 7636 5959/5905
www.biolab.co.uk

Genova Diagnostics Europe
Parkgate House
356 West Barnes Lane
New Malden
Surrey KT3 6NB
Tel +44 (0)20 8336 7750

www.gdx.uk.net

Supplier for nystatin powder

NB: Most patients prefer to put nystatin powder into standard gelatine capsules as its doesn't taste too good.

Courtin and Warner Ltd
19 Phoenix Place
Lewes
Sussex BN7 1JX
Tel: +44 (0)1273 480611

How to take nystatin

Safety

Nystatin has an outstanding safety record and has been used by the medical profession for over 55 years since its original discovery. There is virtually no absorption from the gut and thus no systemic side-effects are possible. Nausea and diarrhoea have occasionally been reported when nystatin has been taken in large dosage over prolonged periods, probably due to a local irritating effect on the gut mucosal lining. An indirect side-effect, a Herxheimer reaction, is explained here and in chapter 7. There are no known adverse inter-reactions with any other drugs.

How to take nystatin

The powder is usually dispersed in a vegetable juice (such as V8), to-mato juice or milk/soya milk.

For adults, the normal starting dose is half a level teaspoon per day dispersed in approximately one-third of a glass of milk or juice. This liquid is then taken in four roughly equal doses throughout the day, preferably before food and before bed. The dosage is gradually increased to 2½ level teaspoons per day (see 'Powder' below). In practice, the first pot of powder usually lasts approximately 3½ weeks. The second pot lasts 2–2½ weeks, but when full dosage is attained a pot of powder is consumed in 10 days.

Alternatively, many patients prefer to place the nystatin powder into capsules, which they buy empty and fill themselves; these are available from any pharmacist. One hundred empty capsules should be enough to encapsulate all the powder in one 25 gram pot of nystatin. You should pull apart the empty capsules and put as much powder as possible into both the larger and the smaller sides before then pressing the two sides together. It can take a few minutes to get the hang of this technique, but usually a pot of 100 capsules can be made up in approximately 45 to 55 minutes.

Important note

Please note that although nystatin is also available on prescription from chemists in the form of tablets, these are **not** recommended because:

- the tablets are sugar-coated;
- they contain quite a toxic dye;
- they are substantially more expensive.

Nystatin dosage schedules

Powder

A 5 ml plastic teaspoon is needed for measuring the dosage. The normal starting dose is ½ level teaspoon per day. The teaspoon should be levelled with a knife and excess powder returned to the pot. A ½ level teaspoon can be reasonably well estimated by removing ½ of the powder on the teaspoon with the knife and also returning it to the pot. This ½ level teaspoon can then added to the juice or milk as already described and shaken/stirred to disperse it. It should then be taken at four roughly equal intervals throughout the day, with the dosage gradually increasing. Thus a convenient schedule for adults would be:

Teaspoons per day	Divided into	For
½	4 equal amounts	5 days
¾	4 equal amounts	5 days
1	4 equal amounts	5 days
1¼	4 equal amounts	5 days
1½	4 equal amounts	5 days
1¾	4 equal amounts	5 days
2	4 equal amounts	5 days
2¼	4 equal amounts	5 days
2½	4 equal amounts	some months

Capsules

If self-made capsules are preferred, the idea is to take these spread evenly over the whole day in three or four doses. Thus a convenient schedule for adults would be:

No. of nystatin capsules	am	Lunch	pm	Evening
2 per day for 5 days	1	0	1	0
3 per day for 5 days	1	1	1	0
4 per day for 5 days	1	1	1	1
5 per day for 5 days	1	1	1	2
6 per day for 5 days	2	2	2	0
7 per day for 5 days	1	2	2	2
8 per day for 5 days	2	2	2	2
9 per day for 5 days	3	3	3	0
10 per day for some months	2	2	3	3

Duration

Most patients need to remain on full dosage (2½ teaspoons of powder or 10 capsules per day) for two to four months, although major clinical improvement is usually seen by the time the patient has been on this dosage for a week or two.

Possible reactions to nystatin

The reason for the slow build-up in dosage relates to the possibility of a **Herxheimer reaction**. Nystatin itself, as stated above, is pretty harmless to humans, but as it makes its way through the alimentary canal it effectively kills off any yeast/fungi. Under an electron microscope it can be seen that the yeast cell walls disintegrate when in contact with nystatin. These cells contain an endotoxin called 'Candida toxin', so if large numbers of yeasts are killed, a lot of this toxin is released. The toxin is absorbed from the gut in the normal course of events. Thus, killing large numbers of yeasts can lead to an accentuation of the very symptoms we are seeking to treat – such as bloating, fatigue, depression, and bowel disturbance – if the yeasts are killed off too quickly.

In most patients, the problem is a mild transitory nuisance, but there is the occasional highly sensitive patient where it can cause quite a lot of problems and it may be that in these circumstances the patient will need to change to a different medication.

Dealing with a Herxheimer (die-off) reaction

A common series of events is depicted below:

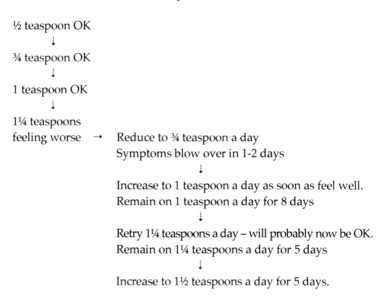

½ teaspoon OK
↓
¾ teaspoon OK
↓
1 teaspoon OK
↓
1¼ teaspoons
feeling worse → Reduce to ¾ teaspoon a day
Symptoms blow over in 1-2 days
↓
Increase to 1 teaspoon a day as soon as feel well.
Remain on 1 teaspoon a day for 8 days
↓
Retry 1¼ teaspoons a day – will probably now be OK.
Remain on 1¼ teaspoons a day for 5 days
↓
Increase to 1½ teaspoons a day for 5 days.

And so on, up to 2½ teaspoons a day. It is obviously possible that further die-off reactions could occur at 1½, 1¾, 2, 2¼ or 2½ teaspoons a day.

Exactly the same reaction can happen whether you are taking nystatin in powder or capsule form and the manner of dealing with it should be the same. Be aware that: 1 (self-made) capsule = approximately ¼ level teaspoon of powder.

Although the die-off response is a nuisance and will temporarily prolong the treatment, many people regard it as a good sign in that it is difficult to have any problems with die-off unless you have the *Candida* yeast problem. As such, die-off confirms the diagnosis. People with no *Candida* problem at all can take colossal doses of nystatin without any adverse effect.

References and bibliography

Chapter 1

1. Prentice AM, Jebb SA. Obesity in Britain: glutton or sloth? *British Medical Journal* 1995; 311: 437-439.

Chapter 2

2. Newburgh H. The cause of obesity. *JAMA* 1931; 23: 1659-1663.

3. Greenwood MR, Cleary M. Adipose tissue metabolism and obesity and genetic obesity. In: Bjorntorp, Cairella, Howard (Eds) 1981 75-79

4. Stunkard A, McLaren HM. The results of treatment for obesity: a review of the literature and a report of a series. *Archives of Internal Medicine* 1959; 103(1): 79-85.

Chapter 3

4a. Grant EC. Food allergies and migrane. *Lancet* 1979; 1(8123): 966-969.

Chapter 4

5. Rinkel HJ. The role of food allergy in internal medicine. *Annals of Allergy* 1944; 2: 115-124.

6. Kennedy GC. The central nervous regulation of calorie balance. *Proceedings of the Nutrition Society* 1961; 20: 58-64.

Brostoff J, Gamlin L. *The Complete Guide to Food Allergy and Intolerance.* 4th edition. Quality Health Books, 2008.

Brostoff J, Challacombe SJ. *Food Allergy and Intolerance.* WB Saunders, 2002. (This is the medical textbook on the subject)

Hare F. *The Food Factor in Disease.* Longman: 1905.

Mackarness R. *Eat Fat and Grow Slim.* Fontana: 1957, 1976

Mackarness R. *Not All in the Mind.* Pan: 1976

Mackarness R. *Chemical Victims.* Pan: 1980.

Randolph TG, Moss R. *An Alternative Approach to Allergies.* Harper Perennial, 1990

Chapter 6

7. Mansfield JR, Burrell MJ et al. Treatment of equine allergic diseases with allergy neutralization: A field study. *Journal of Nutritional and Environmental Medicine* 1998; 8: 329-334.

8. Miller JB. A double-blind study of food extract in injection therapy. *Annals of Allergy* 1977; 38(3): 185-191.

9. Rea WJ. Elimination of oral food challenge reactions by injection of food extracts. *Archives of Otolaryngology* 1984; 110: 248-252.

10. O'Shea JA, Seymour FP. A double-blind study of children with hyperkinetic syndrome treated with multi-allergen extract sublingually. *Journal of Learning Disability* 1981; 14 (4): 189-191.

11. Schiff BM. Broncho-provocation blocked by neutralisation therapy. 1983 *Journal of Allergy and Clinical Immunology* 1983; 71: 92.

12. Brostoff J, Scadding G. Low-dose sublingual therapy in patients with allergic rhinitis due to housedust mite. *Clinical Allergy* 1986; 16: 483-491.

13. Radcliffe MJ, Brostoff J. Allergen specific low-dose immunotherapy in perennial allergic rhinitis: a double-blind placebo-controlled cross-over study. *Journal of Investigational Allergology and Clinical Immunology* 1996; 6(4): 242-247.

14. Finn R. A clinical trial of low-dose desensitization and environmental control. *Clinical Ecology* 1988; 4(2): 75-76.

15. King DS. Can allergic exposure provoke psychological symptoms? A double-blind test. *Biological Psychiatry* 1981; 16: 3-17.

16. Lehman CW. A double-blind study of sublingual provocative food testing. *Annals of Allergy* 1980; 45: 144-149.

17. King WP et al. Provocative neutralization: a two-part study. Part I – The intracutaneous provocative food test: a multi-centre comparison study. *Otolaryngology, Head and Neck Surgery* 1988; 99(3): 263-271.

18. King WP et al. Provocative neutralization: a two-part study. Part II – Subcutaneous neutralisation therapy: a multi-centre comparison study. *Otolaryngology Head and Neck Surgery* 1988; 99(3): 272-277.

Chapter 7

There are literally thousands of clinical papers appertaining to *Candida* in numerous medical conditions, but none specifically relating to weight problems. There have, however, been a lot of books written on the subject. The best ones, in my opinion, are:

Crook WG. *The Yeast Connection Handbook.* Square One Publishing: 2008.

Trowbridge MD, Walker M. *The Yeast Syndrome*. Bantam: 1988.

Truss O. *The Missing Diagnosis* Out of print: 1985.

Yudkin J. *Pure White and Deadly*. Penguin: 1988, 2012.

Chapter 8

19. O'Reilly DS. Thyroid function tests: time for a reassessment. *British Medical Journal* 2000; 320: 1332-1334.

Durrant-Peatfield B. *Your Thyroid and How to Keep it Healthy*. Hammersmith Press Ltd: 2006.

Chapter 9

20. Richard JL. Coronary risk factors: the French paradox. *Archives de Mal Coeur Vaiss* 1987; 80: Spec No 17-21.

21. Hauswirth CB et al. High omega-3 fatty acid content in Alpine cheese: the basis for an Alpine paradox. *Circulation* 2004; 109(1): 103-107.

22. Serra-Majeml et al. Could changes in diet explain changes in coronary artery disease mortality in Spain: the Spanish paradox. *American Journal of Clinical Nutrition* 1995; 61(6): Supp 1351-1359.

23. Keys A. Coronary heart disease in seven countries. *Circulation* 1970; 41(4S1): 1-211.

24. Anitschow N. On variations in the rabbit aorta experimental cholesterol feeding. *Bietre Path Anat u allgem Path* 1913; 56: 379.

25. Herrick JB. Clinical features of sudden obstruction of the coronary arteries. *JAMA* 1912; LIX(23): 2015-2022.

26. Howard BV et al. Low-fat dietary pattern and risk of cardio-vascular disease. (The Women's Health Initiative Randomized Controlled Dietary Modification Trial). *JAMA* 2006; 295(6): 655-666.

27. Leosdottir M et al. Dietary fat intake and early mortality patterns – data from the Malmö Diet and Cancer Study. *Journal of Internal Medicine* 2005; 258(2): 153-165.

28. Frantz ID et al. Test of effect of lipid lowering by diet on cardiovascular risk. The Minnesota Coronary Survey. *Arterio, Thrombo and Vascular Biology* 1989; 9: 129-135.

29. Multiple Risk Factor Trial Research Group. Multiple risk factor intervention trial. Risk factor changes and mortality results. *JAMA* 1982; 248(12): 1465-1477.

30. Stallones RA. Mortality and the multiple risk factor intervention trial. *American Journal of Epidemiology* 1983; 117(6): 647-650.

31. Meittinen M et al. Effect of cholesterol-lowering diet on mortality from coronary heart disease and other causes. *Lancet* 1972; 300(7782): 835-838.

Campbell GD, Cleave TL. *Diabetes, Coronary Thrombosis and the Saccharine Disease*. John Wright: 1966.

Taubes G. *The Diet Delusion*. Vermilion: 2009.

Chapter 10

32. Kekwik A, Pawan GL. Metabolic study in human obesity with iso calorie diets. *Metabolism: Clinical and Experimental* 1957; 6(5): 447-460.

33. Benoit FL et al. Changes in body composition during weight reduction in obesity. *Annals of Internal Medicine* 1965; 63(4): 604-612.

34. Reaven GM. Banting lecture 1988: Role of insulin resistance in human disease. *Diabetes* 1988; 37(12): 1595-1607.

35. Reaven GM et al. Carbohydrate intolerance and hyperlipemia in patients with myocardial infarction without known diabetes

mellitus. *Journal of Clinical Endocrinology and Metabolism* 1963; 23: 1013-1023.

36. Abbasi F et al. High carbohydrate diets, triglyceride rich lipoproteins and coronary artery disease risk. *American Journal of Cardiology* 2000; 85(1): 45-48.

37. Sharman MJ et al. A ketogenic diet favourably affects serum biomarkers for cardiovascular disease in normal weight men. *Human Nutrition and Metabolism* 2002; 1879-1885.

38. Westman EC et al. Effect of 6 month adherence to a very low carbohydrate diet program. 2002 *American Journal of Medicine* 2002; 113(1): 30-36.

39. Foster GD et al. A randomized trial of a low carbohydrate diet for obesity. *New England Journal of Medicine* 2003; 348: 2082-2090.

Agatston A. *The South Beach Diet*. Rodale Press: 2003.

Atkins RC. *Dr Atkins' New Diet Revolution*. Vermilion: 1972, 2003.

Banting W. *A letter on corpulence addressed to the public.* 1863 (Re-issued by Cosimo Classics: 2005).

Cordain L. *The Paleo Diet*. John Wiley: 2010.

Dukan P. *The Dukan Diet*. Hodder: 2000, 2010.

Eades MR, Eades MD, Deans M. *Protein Power*. Bantam 1996, 1998.

Groves B. *Trick and Treat*. Hammersmith Press: 2008.

Holford P. *The Low GL Bible*. Piatkus: 2009.

Stewart L. *Sugar Busters*. Vermilion: 1998.

Stillman IM, Baker SS. *The Doctor's Quick Weight Loss Diet*. 1968.

Taller H. *Calories Don't Count*. Simon: 1961.

Tarnower H, Baker SS, Delvin. *The Complete Scarsdale Medical Diet*. Bantam: 1978, 2003.

Yudkin J. *The Slimming Business*. Penguin: 1962, 1970.

Chapter 11

40. Davies S et al. Age related decreases in chromium levels in 51,665 hair, sweat and serum samples from 40,872 patients: implications for the prevention of cardiovascular disease and type II diabetes. *Metabolism* 1997; 46(5): 469-473.

41. Boyle E et al. Chromium depletion in the pathogenesis of diabetes and atherosclerosis. *South Medical Journal* 1997; 70(12): 1449-1453.

42. Mertz W. Chromium in human nutrition: a review. *Journal of Nutrition* 1993; 123: 626-633.

43. Newman HA et al. Low chromium levels in the aorta are found to correlate with coronary heart disease: Serum chromium and angiographically determined coronary artery disease. *Clinical Chemistry* 1978; 24: 541-544.

44. Vollset SE et al. Plasma total homocysteine and cardiovascular and noncardiovascular mortality: the Hordaland Study. *American Journal of Clinical Nutrition* 2001; 74(1): 130-136.

45. Wald DS, Morris JK, Morris JK. Homocysteine and cardiovascular disease: evidence of causality from a meta analysis. *British Medical Journal* 2002; 325(7374): 1202.

46. Ellis FM, McKully KS. Prevention of myocardial infarction by vitamin B6. *Research Communication Molecular Pathology and Pharmacology* 1995; 89(2): 208-220.

McCully KS. *The Homocysteine Revolution*. McGraw-Hill: 1999.

Holford P, Braly J. *The H Factor*. Piatkus Books: 2003.

Chapter 12

47. Coombes R. Trans fats: chasing a global ban. *British Medical Journal* 2011; 343: (d5567) 506-509.

Mansfield J. *Avoidable Death*. Littlehampton Book Services: 1970.

Chapter 13

48. Thompson JL et al. Effects of diet and diet plus exercise programs on resting metabolic rate: A meta-analysis. *IJSNEM* 1996; 6(1): 41-61.

49. Donnelly JE et al. Effects of a very-low-calorie diet and physical-training regimens on body composition and resting metabolic rate in obese females. *American Journal of Clinical Nutrition* 1991; 54: 56-61.

50. Manson JE et al. A prospective study of walking as compared with vigorous exercise in the prevention of coronary heart disease in women. *New England Journal of Medicine* 1999; 341(9): 650-658.

Chapter 15

51. Nemetz P et al. Recent trends in the prevalence of coronary disease: a population based autopsy study of non-natural deaths. *Archives of Internal Medicine* 2008; 168(3): 264-270.

Index